I0449088

# MESSAGES
## FROM AN ILLNESS

### DEEPENING FAITH THROUGH CANCER

### RUTH BANKESTER SKAGGS

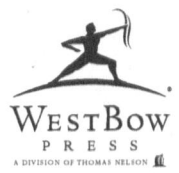

WestBow
PRESS
A DIVISION OF THOMAS NELSON

Copyright © 2013 Ruth Bankester Skaggs.

All rights reserved. No part of this book may be used or reproduced by any means, graphic, electronic, or mechanical, including photocopying, recording, taping or by any information storage retrieval system without the written permission of the publisher except in the case of brief quotations embodied in critical articles and reviews.

All Scriptures referred to are from *The New Oxford Annotated Bible, New Revised Standard Version with the Apocrypha, 3rd ed.*

WestBow Press books may be ordered through booksellers or by contacting:

WestBow Press
A Division of Thomas Nelson
1663 Liberty Drive
Bloomington, IN 47403
www.westbowpress.com
1-(866) 928-1240

Because of the dynamic nature of the Internet, any web addresses or links contained in this book may have changed since publication and may no longer be valid. The views expressed in this work are solely those of the author and do not necessarily reflect the views of the publisher, and the publisher hereby disclaims any responsibility for them.

Any people depicted in stock imagery provided by Thinkstock are models, and such images are being used for illustrative purposes only.

Certain stock imagery © Thinkstock.

ISBN: 978-1-4497-9166-7 (sc)
ISBN: 978-1-4497-9167-4 (hc)
ISBN: 978-1-4497-9165-0 (e)

Library of Congress Control Number: 2013906965

Printed in the United States of America.

WestBow Press rev. date: 5/20/2013

In memory of my parents

Gertrude Ganus Bankester

and

Artemas Bankester

# ABOUT THE AUTHOR

FOR MANY YEARS RUTH SKAGGS had a private practice in Atlanta, Georgia, as a licensed professional counselor, music psychotherapist, and registered expressive arts therapist. In 2003 she closed her practice in Atlanta and returned to the Alabama Gulf Coast, her birthplace. She now teaches piano in Daphne. She is a communicant of St. Paul's Episcopal Church in Daphne, where she is a lay eucharistic minister.

She has two sons and two grandsons.

Skaggs is the author of *Finishing Strong: Treating Chemical Addictions with Music and Imagery* and *Music: Keynote of the Human* Spirit. She has compiled a compact disc, *Music For Healing I*. Further information may be obtained at www.ruthskaggs.com.

# ACKNOWLEDGMENTS

I F I WERE A POET I would write an ode to public libraries. They are an underused gift from our governments big and small. Anne Morris, reference librarian at Daphne Public Library, with the heart of a true librarian helped me cheerfully with research and obtaining articles and books through the interlibrary loan system.

The Reverend Albert Kennington and The Reverend Dr. Richard Schmidt were willing readers and made valuable comments. Peggy Jeffery was an in-the-field reader as she read and gave helpful comments while undergoing treatments for cancer. Emily Rome, who in another life edited manuals for the U.S. Air Force, gave enormous help in organizing the content and clarifying some otherwise obtuse thoughts.

Thanks to my great medical team: my primary physician, Dr. Suzanne Tormoen, and her nurse, Elizabeth Johnston; my oncologist, Dr. Michael Meshad; and my surgeon, Dr. Charles Smith. Without you I wouldn't be here. Thanks to all of the wonderful and always cheerful oncology nurses and staff at the Southern Cancer Center. I don't know how you can stay so positive and upbeat when you're dealing with life and death every day.

Thanks to Dave Hale, who takes care of my computer and internet challenges. And many thanks to the friends who encouraged me throughout the writing of this book, especially Jean Palmer, Liana Carey, Carol Jones, Ken McNamara, Caron Richards, Jean Erwin, and Frances Kimbrough. If I've left anyone out, it's because of an imperfect memory, not a lack of gratitude.

# TABLE OF CONTENTS

# INTRODUCTION

MY DIAGNOSIS OF CANCER SHOOK me to the core. How could this have happened? My annual physical examination only a few months earlier had shown that I was in good health. In fact, I had been remarkably healthy all my life. I couldn't believe my diagnosis of non-Hodgkin's lymphoma. I couldn't understand what had happened to change my body so quickly.

In their 2011 report, the American Cancer Society (ACS) predicted that more than fifteen hundred people would die of cancer per day during that year. According to the ACS, cancer is the second most common cause of death in the United States, exceeded only by heart disease. Cancer accounts for nearly one of every four deaths in this wealthy, privileged country we live in. It is little wonder that a diagnosis of cancer brings anxiety to the persons who have been diagnosed with it, and to their loved ones. Everyone knows someone who has, or has had, cancer. Everyone knows someone who has survived cancer and others who have not.

Since I received the diagnosis of cancer I have learned from the many people I know who are, or have been, cancer patients that my initial responses were not uncommon. Shock and disbelief are common first responses of all people who are suddenly faced with a life-threatening illness. After the initial shock, however, the responses people have are many and varied. There is no template for dealing with the onset of such a disease.

Although there are books and articles that may offer help in dealing with our disease, there are no guaranteed recipes, rules, or maps. Each cancer is unique and deeply personal. No one has ever been inside someone else's cancer. No one has been inside my cancer, except me. There can be no one set of guidelines to direct us through the new and untried experience of having a toxic disease. There is no global positioning system (GPS) to keep us from getting confused and lost on this journey.

For many years I have practiced meditation and contemplative prayer. When I received the diagnosis of cancer I immediately knew it was far more than a medical diagnosis. I realized it was a barometer of my mental, emotional, and spiritual life. Something besides my physical health was out of order and needed to be made right. I believed this was God's way of getting my attention so that God could teach me something I had not learned, something I had neither seen nor heard in spite of many opportunities to do so.

As soon as I opened myself to the larger purpose of my illness, I began to receive messages during my prayer times. Many passages in the Judeo-Christian Scriptures spoke to me in ways that were piercingly relevant to my new condition. Almost daily, revelations and guidance came to me. Since I'm not a theologian, my responses to the Scriptures aren't theological interpretations. Rather, I think they are more akin to those of the people for whom the authors of the Bible were writing—ordinary people with ordinary lives and universal human needs. I kept all of the revelations in a journal. That journal gradually expanded and unfolded, experience by experience, until it became the basis for this book.

My belief in the power of prayer has been reinforced over and over throughout my life. It has helped me in moving through personal struggles and making difficult decisions. When I became the receiver of intercessory prayers, my concept of prayer expanded. Prayer took on new meaning as I felt the intentionality of God's caring people focused specifically on my healing. As I experienced prayer in a different way I began to look into studies made on the effectiveness of prayer. I have shared the findings from my study of prayer, religion, and spirituality in general and, specifically, as they relate to cancer.

My training and experience in the use of expressive arts therapies for bringing healing and transformation to others helped me enormously in the difficult days of chemotherapy and other aspects of the illness. With a degree in church music and a strong calling to use music in a more direct healing capacity, I had accomplished the long process of a career change some years earlier.

After earning a graduate degree in psychology I became a licensed professional counselor. I trained in the Bonny Method of Guided Imagery and Music (BMGIM), a remarkable depth psychotherapy that uses carefully selected music as the vehicle for healing and change. In addition I became a registered expressive arts therapist through the International Expressive Arts Therapy Association.

All of the healing modalities that I had studied and practiced professionally—music, imagery, and other expressive arts—were natural additions to my cancer treatment. Because I had witnessed them as being profoundly helpful to the clients in my private practice, I realized how beneficial they would be to me and other people who have cancer. In these chapters I describe my use of these healing arts in my recovery and speculate on their role in my unpredictably early remission. I have attempted to explain them clearly enough so that cancer patients, or patients of any serious or life-threatening illness, can use them in their own healing.

My deep faith in God and the communion with my church family at St. Paul's Episcopal Church in Daphne, Alabama, also were essential in sustaining me and keeping me from getting lost. The support of my immediate family and my rather large extended family provided an unwavering anchor that would not let me weaken in my commitment to being a fully active participant in my healing process. The loving concerns of family and friends brought me a feeling of responsibility to do my part in getting well.

I began writing this book when I was in partial remission and continuing treatment in the form of a maintenance drug. I may have to live with this drug for a long time, but I am grateful for the spiritual growth this cancer has provided me. There have been many teaching moments I might not have experienced but for this illness. I trust in God's mysterious ways of bringing things to fruition.

I have not attempted to give cancer patients a tutorial on how to navigate through their cancer. My hope is that my experiences will offer perspectives that will encourage them to take hold of their healing journey, call on God for guidance, and find the teaching in their own illness. As long as we have a dreadful disease, why not grab hold of whatever good we can get from it?

As Rabbi Harold Kushner explained, we can't always control what happens to us, but we can control how we respond to painful events in our lives. He asks, "How can we turn all the painful experiences of our lives into birth pangs or into growing pains?" By being aware and committed to finding meaning in pain and illness, we can find what the illness does to us. What does it reveal about our relationship to God and God's people? What revelations about ourselves will unfold? Who will we become because of the illness? How will it change us?

In the field of counseling I learned that every encounter has the potential for changing us in some way, though the change may be small, subtle, and slow to be revealed. An encounter such as a conversation with a friend or stranger, or with an event, tragedy, or illness can change our attitudes, understanding, and responses to life. My encounter with cancer has the potential to change who I am and who I will be in the remaining years of my life. My hope is that I will be a better person, no matter the outcome of the treatments.

"Who am I, O Lord God, and what is my house, that you have brought me thus far?" (2 Samuel 7:18)

I dare to hope that, in the words of Teresa of Avila, the sixteenth century saint, "God will take this insignificant contribution of ours (mine) and unite it with his greatness, rendering it with such value that . . . his efforts and ours become one."

# { 1 }

# A LIFE-CHANGING JOLT

"**P**ATHOLOGY SUGGESTING LYMPHOMA." THE REPORT from my computerized tomography (CT) scan left me reeling. From two enlarged lymph nodes I could see and feel, I knew it must be lymphoma, or something that was equally bad news. Questions flashed through my mind. What will this mean for me? How advanced is this disease? What will I have to do? Can I continue to live my life in a reasonably normal way? Will I have to go through immobilizing, debilitating treatments? I have known people with cancer. Some of them were very sick. Some didn't make it. The lack of answers in this initial stage made life seem almost surreal. A call to my sons to tell them about the scan results left them in similar states. What was going to happen?

The report was hard for me to absorb, in particular, because of my environmentally conscious lifestyle. As a volunteer environmental educator teaching in schools, I had independently engaged in a lot of research on how the environment affects our health. I had learned that research conducted by universities and independent environmental organizations revealed the presence

1

of chemicals harmful to humans in many personal care products and commercial cleaning products. I also found there is very little governmental oversight on many of these products.

As a result of this research I eliminated all of those harmful chemicals from my life some years ago, and have used only products that contain natural, nonharmful ingredients. My shelves are stocked with large containers of white distilled vinegar and baking soda, as well as other ingredients for safe cleaning and personal care use. I have maintained fairly healthy eating habits, without being unreasonable about it. In spite of all my efforts to live a healthy lifestyle I was struck by cancer. It seemed unfair.

In a conversation with my primary care doctor, Suzanne Tormoen, I received details of what was ahead: a biopsy to determine with a certainty that I had lymphoma, tests to determine what kind of lymphoma I had, then on to an oncologist (how scary that word was) to plan a treatment for me.

I had almost no energy the day after the scan report. I slept a lot. I finally realized that being so shaken about the report had sapped my energy. It was such a relief to learn this wasn't a permanent state—at least not right away.

On the second post-diagnosis day, a Sunday, I still felt very tired but decided to go to church, promising myself that this thing wasn't going to intimidate me. Going to church and singing in the choir, both routine things for me to do on a Sunday, restored some sense of normalcy and helped me to gain a little energy.

On the third day I followed my usual morning routine of Scripture study from the Judeo-Christian Bible: meditation on the Scriptures, prayers for people and matters of concern, followed by contemplative prayer. A conversation with God is often a part of this practice. When I reach the state of quiet that is the goal of contemplative prayer I'm simply listening to what God wants to say to me. The Scriptures I read are from the lectionary in the Book of Common Prayer of the Episcopal Church. A Catholic friend told me that my daily practice is called *lectio divina* in her religion, something I didn't know, although I have been practicing it for years. I like the name *lectio* divina—divine reading. It is a way of praying with the Scriptures that involves reading, reflection, meditation, contemplative prayer, and silently waiting for God. I will discuss more about the practice of *lectio divina* in Chapter 3. Also on that third day I remembered a Scripture that had strongly influenced me years before. Looking it up in the concordance, I found it in l Corinthians 10:13:

> ... *God is faithful, and he will not let you be tested beyond your strength, but with the testing he will also provide the way out so that you will be able to endure it.*

What a comforting promise! Every challenge is accompanied by the help needed to get through it.

A biopsy a few weeks later confirmed: non-Hodgkin's lymphoma, stage 3. Later, during my first appointment with my oncologist, the doctor told me that stage 4 is the most advanced stage. This disease had advanced considerably with no visible signs until a few months prior to discovery. A swollen right foot was the only symptom that took me to my physician and eventually led to this diagnosis. A scan showed that I now had multiple tumors throughout my body.

Non-Hodgkin's lymphoma is cancer that begins in the cells of the immune system, the system that fights infections and other diseases. Each year more than sixty-three thousand Americans learn they have non-Hodgkin's lymphoma. Although it can occur in young people, the chance of developing this disease goes up with age. Most people with non-Hodgkin's lymphoma are over sixty.

After reading the possible causes of lymphoma to see whether I had done, or not done, something to cause this disease, I arrived at one cause relevant to me: aging. Ah, I thought. That is totally out of my control. I could have done nothing to avoid that.

As I was reflecting on the "why me?" question, another question popped into my mind: "Why *not* me?" I immediately dismissed that debate. I didn't want to expend energy trying to find answers to questions for which only God knows the answer. I needed all my physical and mental energies to get on with the task of healing.

We who live on the Gulf Coast are taught that if we're unfortunate enough to get caught in a rip current while swimming in the Gulf, the safest and wisest thing to do is to swim *with* the current, allowing it to carry us out farther until it loses its strength. Powerful rip currents are too strong even for good swimmers. Fighting a rip current, trying to swim against it, leaves the swimmer exhausted. Drowning often follows. However, when going *with* the current until its strength weakens, the swimmer can then swim parallel to the shore until a safe spot can be found to swim back to shore. The term "going with the flow" takes on new meaning in this metaphor.

On one of my sickest days, when I could barely lift my head from the pillow, I remembered this analogy. It allowed me to move *with* the experience, not giving up but using the power of the surge to carry me until it ran its course. Angrily fighting against it or giving in to despair would have rendered me helpless.

While fighting against cancer can be unproductive, a spirit of cooperation along with treatments, good medical advice, and

God's guidance can be empowering. It would make me a fully participating member of the team whose goal was to help me to heal. Experiencing it as if I were a pilgrim on a journey with wide-open eyes, open mind, and open heart could lead me safely back to shore and whatever awaited me there.

In John 9:1-4 there is a story of Jesus healing a blind man. In answer to his disciples' question about the cause of the man's blindness Jesus shifted the emphasis from the cause to the purpose. Jesus said, "We must work the works of him who sent me."

I knew there was a larger purpose at work, and there were meanings to be gleaned from my illness. God does nothing by accident. He is in everything, including cancer. Side by side with God's promise to provide the way through this cancer was *my* promise to search for the hidden meanings and to allow them to be revealed so that I could learn what truths God was trying to teach me.

I prayed:

> *In spite of living a healthy life—eliminating harmful chemicals, trying to make a small footprint on earth—I have this awful infection throughout my body. I can't comprehend it, but I want to follow your will, Lord. It's so hard going through this, but I know there's something you want me to learn from it. You certainly have my attention. Give me eyes to see, ears to hear, and a mind and heart to comprehend.*

When Mary, who was to become the mother of Jesus, was visited by the angel Gabriel and given the shocking news of her pregnancy, her response was, "Here am I, the servant of the Lord;

let it be with me according to your word" (Luke 1:38). She was still a virgin, betrothed to Joseph. The implications of her conception must have been enormous and frightening. Here she was, a young teenager engaged to a man who believed her to be a virgin. He could have broken the engagement and left her to be shamed and ostracized by her religious community.

Biblical scholars believe Mary to have been around fourteen at the time of the angel's pronouncement. Fourteen was marriageable age in those times, yet Mary was still an inexperienced girl, not a grown woman. Did she go to her mother for help in sorting out this remarkable event? For help in what she should do? To find out if her mother would be ashamed of her pregnancy? How did she break the news to Joseph? Did she ask him for advice?

The Scriptures tell us virtually nothing about the time between Gabriel's message and Mary's response. They indicate that her response was immediate. We can only speculate that she went through some agonizing, soul-searching thoughts about God's mandate and what it would mean for her. Yet she accepted it with complete obedience to God's plan for her.

Figuratively speaking, I've walked across hot coals more than once. I believed I could do it again. I felt I could accept the challenge of cancer. I've faced many challenges, including several mid-life crises—divorce, single-parenting two boys in their early teens, and making a career change. Navigating those drastic life-changes was on-the-job training, pure and simple. Nowhere are there classes that adequately prepare us for such changes. I survived reasonably intact, though not without some soul-wrenching struggles. Still, even with the endurance and emotional strength I had gained from meeting these challenges, I wasn't sure I could face this new test as fully as Mary met hers. Could I not only surrender to God's will but also sing "My soul magnifies the Lord" (Luke 1:46) with the passion and joy and acceptance heard in Mary's song? Could I praise God as chemotherapy drugs dripped through me?

The patriarch Abraham was almost one hundred years old and childless when God promised him he would be the father of us all. His wife, Sarah, was many years beyond childbearing ability. Amazed as Abraham must have been at what was promised him, still he put his trust in God. When the evangelist Paul spoke of Abraham many years later he said, ". . . he grew strong in his faith as he gave glory to God" (Romans 4:20).

I marvel that both Mary and Abraham had such faith in the unknown. Neither had any idea of the outcome of God's promises. The power of God's plan had consequences far beyond anything either of them could have imagined.

I wondered if I could grow into the faith and trust shown by Mary and Abraham. Although I had a deep faith in God's power, I have wanted more. I have wanted to have the faith that *moves mountains.* I wondered if God's purpose in this illness was to guide me toward surrendering with complete trust to God's plan for me. And to do it while praising God.

I realized I had to begin with surrendering and letting God guide me through it—the same way Mary and Abraham were led when they surrendered to God's will.

Surrendering to God's plan brought a new sense of what discipleship means. I found that being a true disciple demanded that I use all of my resources, my life experiences, all of the gifts I have been given through the years to meet this challenge. Much of my life to this point had been preparation for this test.

From the psalmist I read, "But I trust in you, O Lord; I say, 'You are my God.' My times are in your hand" (Psalm 31:14-15a).

I prayed:

> *I do trust in you, Lord. I know I'm in your hands. Help me to remember always to glorify you no matter how tough this gets. Glorifying you through this illness appears to be your way of testing me. If I meet this test successfully, I believe my faith will draw closer to the faith that moves mountains.*

At this time in my life my sons are grown and gone, with families of their own. I have been living alone enough years to have fine-tuned the art of self-sufficiency. I have often called on God for help and guidance, but I forgot that God works through his people. When something needed to be done I rarely asked for help from family or friends. My philosophy was to do it myself, pay to have it done, or leave it undone. Little did I know that my prideful self-sufficiency would soon be shattered by a knockout punch. In the following chapters I tell about my humbling experiences as I waded through the many difficulties of cancer and its treatment.

# { 2 }

# UNCHARTED TERRITORY

THE NEXT STEP WAS TO see an oncologist. Before that happened, though, I had another shock. Dr. Tormoen sent me to Thomas Medical Center to have another CT scan. I was still feeling very healthy and planning to have lunch with a friend following the scan. The technicians administering the scan commented that I didn't look sick nor did I act sick.

To my great distress, the radiologist reading the scan found blood clots on both sides of my lungs. After consulting with Dr. Tormoen the technicians called an ambulance to transport me to Thomas Hospital where I would be admitted. I was feeling so good I couldn't understand why the technicians and ambulance attendants wouldn't let me drive myself to the hospital nor even let me walk from the exam room to the ambulance.

Later, when I saw the diagnosis, "severe pulmonary embolism," I began to understand the seriousness of the situation. My healthy life hadn't prepared me for what was happening now.

My two brothers who live nearby, Merrill and Edward, were notified. My two sons, both living out of state, were notified, as well as Father Thack Dyson, rector of St. Paul's. My brothers and

Father Thack were at the hospital soon thereafter. Mark and Chris, my sons, were soon in touch by telephone.

Evan, my grandson, called from college and expressed how worried he was about me. To ease his worries I replied with conviction, "I'm going to do whatever I need to do to get well." If I hadn't yet been committed to getting well, I was now. How could I not be? Jean, a friend who is a retired nurse, told me that with every patient facing difficult medical procedures, there is a moment when a mental button is pushed, the button that decides whether the patient will strive to live or let go and deteriorate or die. My sweet grandson's concern was my button. I was going to follow every doctor's order, go through every necessary procedure, and focus all of my energy on getting well.

Merrill and his wife, Peggy, retrieved my car from the Medical Center and put it in my garage. They also got some personal articles from the house that I would need. I quickly realized that with a serious illness such as this I needed the support and help of an entire squadron of family, friends, and relatives.

A comedic episode lightened our tension. When Merrill and Peggy went to my house to get the requested articles, I had left my security system on. They didn't carry the code with them, but Merrill knew that the code was a familiar word spelled out in numbers on a telephone keypad. When they entered the house he realized with dismay that the alarm keypad had no letters on it, only numbers. While the alarm was ticking away, they searched frantically for my telephone to retrieve the letters in the code. They couldn't find it soon enough, and the alarm started blaring. After quickly retrieving the things I wanted, they were leaving the house just as a police officer drove up. Caught red-handed! The worst scenario would have been for the officer to arrest them. Instead, he took one look at this frantic, aging couple driving a late-model car, with my house keys and a few personal articles in their hands, and he apparently believed their story. When they told me what happened I could see, in my fertile imagination, the officer trying to maintain a passive face while resisting an instinct to roll his eyes.

I remained in the hospital for three days until the blood clots decreased, then was sent home with an order for a daily dose of Coumadin, a blood thinner.

On my first visit with Dr. Michael Meshad, the oncologist I had chosen, he gave me more complete information from the biopsy and scan. "This is non-Hodgkin's lymphoma, B cell, stage 3," he said. "B cell is easier to treat than T cell." Well, that's hopeful, I thought.

While examining my body for swollen lymph glands, he found tumors in multiple places. What was particularly worrisome was either a markedly enlarged spleen or, perhaps, a large mass of lymph nodes behind the spleen. He expressed concern that they could eventually block my kidneys or other organs and suggested that we begin treatment the following week.

Treatment would be a combination of chemotherapy and immunotherapy (Rituxan) given in one intravenous treatment, once every three weeks. He predicted that after four to six treatments the lymph glands would be decreased enough in size that we could cease the chemotherapy treatments and continue with Rituxan once every two months until the cancer was in full remission, perhaps in two years. My body responded to treatment much more quickly than his prediction, as I describe later in this chapter.

Dr. Meshad told me that if the lymphoma hadn't been so advanced we could treat it with Rituxan only, but "there isn't time to do that." If you've never been told that your clock is ticking rapidly it will be difficult to comprehend the shock I felt.

Dr. Meshad added that lymphoma isn't typically cured; it's "controlled." More hope came when he added, "Old people do much better with treatments than young people." Well, there are some advantages to getting old, I thought. Not a lot, but some.

"People your age don't often experience nausea and vomiting," he continued. He added that I would have fatigue, be more susceptible to infections, and would lose my hair. He seemed very certain about what would happen, and it turned out he was correct.

He filled me with relief when he said, "We need to make sure that each treatment makes you better, not worse. If a treatment makes you terribly sick I won't do that one again." Later, I remembered what he had said when the side effects from the first treatment were so horrendous I didn't know whether I could endure another one like it. I called him and asked if we could adjust the treatments. "Of course," he answered. "I don't want you to go through that again."

True to his word, in the next treatment Dr. Meshad eliminated one of the chemotherapy drugs and the following injection of Neulaste that was aimed at restoring the white blood cells depleted by the chemotherapy drugs. What a difference! The side effects from the next two treatments were very unpleasant, but more tolerable.

In that first visit Dr. Meshad spoke with a strong, sincere conviction that the treatment would have a positive outcome. He convinced me. I knew with certainty that I had chosen the right oncologist. Later, when I reflected on that visit I remembered some of my earlier research which shed light on Dr. Meshad's positive talk:

> *Robert Ornstein and David Sobel, in their studies of self-healing mechanisms in the long history of medical treatments, have found that it wasn't the specific* <u>*treatment*</u> *that brought the cure. It has been, rather, the* <u>*belief*</u> *in the treatment and the healer. Physicians can give a message that the illness is hopeless, and treatment will involve much pain. Or they can communicate a positive attitude through their choice of words, voice tone, and body language. Ornstein and Sobel also found that the message given with the treatment even influences how rapidly the treatment takes effect. It is important to choose doctors who understand how powerful their influence is on the belief system of the patient and who will use that power to effect a positive outcome.*

I don't know whether Dr. Meshad was aware of the studies, but he certainly knew what a cancer patient needs. When I was making my choice of an oncologist I learned that Dr. Meshad had been a cancer patient himself. Through that experience he had learned firsthand the emotional needs of a person walking through cancer.

Between my initial appointment with Dr. Meshad and the first treatment the following week, I had to have a positron emission tomography (PET) scan to determine the full extent of the disease. Also, I had to be examined by a cardiologist to determine the health of my heart and undergo surgery to get a port installed to facilitate the intravenous chemotherapy drugs. My life was filled with appointments, all centered around my illness. There was little time for anything else. My normal life, as I knew it, was gone.

What was before me was uncharted territory. It was scary. In my morning conversations with God, Jesus appeared in my inner vision and told me, "I will lend you my strength."

A church friend, Janice, accompanied me to outpatient surgery to have the port installed. Janice said, "I know what is happening to you is scary, and I'm here to make it less scary." She was with me in the preop room just prior to surgery. My nurse friend Caron had hand-picked my anesthesia nurse, Tricia. Tricia was the perfect choice—calm, steady, comforting, ready to escort me into the operating room. At that moment, Lee (Caron's husband and, also, an anesthesia nurse) popped in to see how I was doing. Janice, Lee, Tricia and I then held hands while Janice prayed over me, moments before I went to never-never land.

Later I realized I had forgotten to call on Jesus for strength! How did I get through it? The insight came immediately, like a hand slap on my forehead. Jesus gave his strength through Janice, Tricia, and Lee. They were conduits for the love, compassion, and comfort of Jesus.

Much later, I reflected on all the help that was given to me throughout my illness. It occurred to me that this kind of group purpose brings to everyone involved a sense of community that is so sadly missing in most of our lives. The value of community of family, community of church, and community of other organizations where people care for one another becomes obvious in times of such need. It is where the Christian "we are one body" principle comes alive. Praying in groups, bringing food, providing transportation for medical appointments are acts of communal outreach that embrace all people—those who think alike, those who don't, church members, and non-church members. I'm certain that these helpers wouldn't vote the same way at the polls or in many other situations. It's the best example I know of how, when a group is focused on a common purpose, unity can work amid diversity. And of how a communal goal can make it possible for us to live peacefully within the one body of Christ.

## FIRST CHEMOTHERAPY TREATMENT

Merrill drove me to the Southern Cancer Center where I was to have all of my chemotherapy treatments. I took with me music programs I had compiled on audiotape, a tape player, head phones, and a pad for journaling. I had compiled the music programs over a period of years for use with the clients in my psychotherapy practice. They were designed to match different moods and different needs to assist clients in making desired changes.

The programs I chose to use that day and with succeeding treatments were those that would best sustain and support me through the multiple emotions I was experiencing. The programs are listed in Appendix D, along with suggestions for other beneficial music. By the end of the series of chemotherapy treatments, my ancient tape player stopped working. Later when I was in remission and taking the maintenance drug every two months I searched for newer music-playing technology. I realized I needed to move into the twenty-first century and update my equipment in the event I should need chemotherapy treatments again. I didn't want to endure chemotherapy without the help of music. Chapter 5 explains more fully the value of music in healing.

When Merrill and I arrived at the cancer center, the first thing I noticed was the open feeling in the building. In the waiting rooms there are comfortable chairs spaced far enough apart to allow quiet conversation. Most impressive, though, are the glass walls that bring the outdoors inside. When I entered the room where the treatments are administered I noticed many reclining chairs placed around the room. These are the chairs for the patients. Each chair has access to a television with a remote.

As in the waiting rooms, the walls in the treatment room were glass from floor to ceiling. Outside are well-kept, beautiful grounds. The view brought a sigh of calm and gratitude from me. For all of the treatments I always chose a chair near a window wall. As the seasons progressed I enjoyed the beauty of magnolias and gardenias in bloom. The bridge between the interior and exterior world seemed almost seamless. My cancer was uniquely mine, but bringing the outside world in helped me to realize that my cancer and I were part of the larger world. We were in God's world, with no boundaries of time or space.

I was told that the first treatment would be quite long. It turned out to be almost six hours. The treatment involved intravenous doses of Benadryl and three chemotherapy drugs, followed by Rituxan, the immunotherapy drug. The Benadryl, administered first, began to make me feel very sleepy, almost drunk. I started listening to the music as soon as the treatment began. I wrote what I was feeling before I had to give in to the sleepiness from the Benadryl. Here is what I wrote in my journal:

*This is scary. I feel a loss of my old self, my old life.*
*All of these chemicals being fed into my body to kill the*
*bad cells along with the good ones is like a yin/yang of*

*bad/good. The medicine is destroying both the bad and good cells so that good cells can reemerge healthy and free of poison.*

*Can my body sustain all of these invasions, all of this destruction? And can it emerge strong and healthy in new life? It's like burning off fields, only to see new plants emerge amid the destruction. What will emerge for me in this new life?*

*There are many political and philosophical differences between me and some of my friends and family members who have stepped up to support and sustain me and give me any help I might need. It seems that at the bottom core of almost everyone there is a living humanity that recognizes and responds to the needs of others. The Holy Spirit clears the pathway and allows us to see beauty in the soul of each. Giving people the opportunity to serve, accompanied by my heartfelt responses of gratitude, allows all of us to experience the deep connectedness among all who are the body of Christ. At the surface level of our consciousness—the level that is absorbed by busyness and clutter—there is division and dissension. At a deeper level—the level that motivates us to love our neighbor—there is unity. The sense of connection that comes as we muddle through the busyness and reach closer to our soul transcends all differences.*

For the first two days following my treatment I didn't feel bad, other than being very tired. On the second day I had an injection of Neulaste, a drug designed to build up the white blood cell count that is diminished by chemotherapy drugs. I thought, This isn't going to be bad at all. I can carry on my life without interruptions.

Day three came in like one of our Gulf Coast hurricanes. I felt as if I had been caught up and pounded by gale-force winds. My bones hurt. Every inch of my body ached and throbbed. I felt as if I had a very bad case of the flu, without the fever. I had no appetite. I could barely function. Although I had antinausea medication I was so sick I couldn't distinguish nausea from my other physical problems. Consequently, one day I vomited several times before I recognized the nausea for what it was, and before the medication I took could take effect. Things got worse every day until they reached a peak about a week after treatment. Although I knew the treatment was very aggressive due to the advanced stage of my lymphoma I hadn't had any idea of what my reactions would be. Since reactions are very individual no one could have accurately predicted what mine would be.

I recognized I needed someone to stay with me. How naïve I had been to think I could do this alone. Merrill stayed with me a day and night. Peggy stayed with me a day and night. My friend Jean E. stayed a couple of days and a night. Joan, who is staff assistant at St. Paul's, stayed a couple of nights. Father Thack came by to see me and said, "Joan is at your disposal. Whatever you need, call her. We're going to get you through this."

Ten days after my first treatment I began to have a turnaround. Joan spent Saturday night with me. On Sunday morning I felt better, but still had no appetite. I told Joan not to fix any breakfast for me. She went on to church. Later I found I was hungry, so I got up and fixed a soft-boiled egg and piece of toast. Soon after, my heart started pounding, and I felt so dizzy I couldn't stand. I went to bed, and the symptoms didn't subside.

Mark called to check on me, and I was too sick to talk to him. I called Joan at church and said, "I need you." She came immediately and called the cancer center. The nurse at the center told me to go to the emergency room at Thomas Hospital. Joan left word with Father Thack, who was still presiding at the service. She drove me to the ER and got me admitted.

Father Thack came to the ER as soon as the service was over. He and Joan helped me through the process of answering all the questions and going through the tests being administered. Father Thack then laid his hand on my head and prayed. I know God's love administered through that calm, beneficent hand has brought comfort to many of us who have experienced it.

Mark had called Merrill to find out what was happening to me. Merrill and Peggy tracked me down, and they arrived at the ER soon after.

At the ER I had many tests, including an EKG. My heart was fine, and the doctor could find nothing that would cause the symptoms I experienced. The symptoms went away not long after I arrived at the ER. I was sent home at the end of the day.

The ER doctor had suspected anxiety as the cause of the symptoms and administered Ativan. After being a licensed professional counselor for many years, however, I knew what anxiety was like. I had experienced no anxiety until the heart pounding and dizziness began. Then, I was decidedly anxious.

Two days later, soon after getting up, I began to experience the same symptoms. This time I knew my heart was fine. I went to bed until the symptoms went away. I contacted Dr. Tormoen to get her help in suggesting foods that would help me build up my strength and immune system. Her list of high-protein foods and drinks was very helpful. For many weeks my refrigerator and shelves were stocked with Gatorade, Ensure Plus, chicken, eggs, ice cream, custard, and cans of tuna fish and clear soup.

My sons and I realized we had to make plans to have someone with me after future treatments. A good friend, Diane, would come from Atlanta and be with me for a week after the second treatment. Mark would be with me after the third treatment, and Chris would come after the fourth one. As it turned out, there wouldn't be a fourth treatment of chemotherapy.

## SECOND CHEMOTHERAPY TREATMENT

Theologian Dietrich Bonhoeffer once commented, "Every Christian must be fully human by bringing God into his whole life, not merely into some spiritual realm." When preparing for my second chemotherapy treatment I took my music, a book, a journal, and God with me. These treatments were now a part of my life and shouldn't be separate from my spiritual activities. Just as God is present in the homilies and the Eucharist on Sunday I wanted to experience God's presence in this new and unpleasant part of my life.

I remembered a passage from Paul's letter to the Romans and reaffirmed it with my own additions (underlined):

> *For I am convinced that neither death, nor life, nor angels, nor rulers, nor things present, nor things to come, nor powers, nor height, nor depth, <u>nor cancer, nor chemotherapy</u>, nor anything else in all creation, will be able to separate me from the love of God in Christ Jesus our Lord* (Romans 8:38-39).

I was committed to bringing my humanness into one whole being with my spiritual nature. Isn't that what Jesus modeled for us? Jesus, being both fully human and fully divine, showed us the way.

God was with me at the cancer center as the strong drugs entered and infiltrated my body. God kept me calm and receptive to the treatment as I accepted that it was a necessary part of my healing.

## THIRD CHEMOTHERAPY TREATMENT

Just before my third chemotherapy treatment, Dr. Meshad examined me and looked at my white blood cell count. His response was, "I'm impressed." And again more deeply, "I'm *impressed*." He couldn't feel a single swollen lymph node in my body, and my white blood cell count was "good." He said instead of a fourth chemotherapy treatment I might be able to go into the remission/ maintenance mode. When I asked how we would know, he said he would send me for another CT scan just prior to the scheduled fourth treatment. The CT scan would show whether I was, indeed, in remission.

I was euphoric! Dr. Meshad had predicted at the beginning that I would need between four and six chemotherapy treatments before I would be "in good enough remission" to go into a maintenance mode. I think Dr. Meshad was as surprised and ecstatic as I was at how quickly my body had responded to the treatments, because he gave me a big hug and a smile. I know he must lose patients in spite of his best efforts. I can only imagine what a sense of accomplishment and pleasure it must give him to know that he has helped someone to overcome the illness—especially ahead of predictions. Although I followed through with the third chemotherapy treatment that day, the strong probability was that I was in partial remission after only two treatments.

Soon after I learned I might be in remission I read in my prayer time:

> *For this reason I bow my knees before the Father . . . I pray that, according to the riches of his glory, he may grant that you may be strengthened in your inner being with power through his Spirit, and that Christ may dwell in your hearts through faith, as you are being rooted and grounded in love. I pray that you may have the power to comprehend, with all the saints, what is the breadth and length and height and depth, and to know the love of Christ that surpasses knowledge, so that you may be filled with all the fullness of God* (Ephesians 3:14-19).

A light turned on in my brain. One of the messages in this passage is about following the will of God, not fighting what was happening, but letting God lead me day by day through this experience. I know that sometimes healing comes through death, and I know that I am going to die someday. When I was first diagnosed I never prayed to live or die. I prayed that God would guide me through this and give me what I needed to meet the challenge, no matter the outcome. I realized that this is the experience of submitting to God's will. I could turn my life over to God and trust in his plan for me, whatever the plan was. In that moment I felt enormous love for and from God.

At church one morning I learned that one of our faithful members had died suddenly. His pleasant face was often visible as he participated in many of our services. I wondered: Did he have any warning, any inkling that his life would quickly be over? Did he have time to put his spiritual life in order? Did he have time to let his family know how much he loved them?

This cancer had been unpleasant and disruptive, changing my normal life into a "new" normal. It surely wasn't something I asked for. Still, when learning of our parishioner's death, I felt grateful that I have had this time to ferret out my spiritual flaws and try to mend them.

Jesus' parable of the ten bridesmaids in Matthew 25 ends with his admonishment, "Keep awake therefore, for you know neither the day nor the hour." In this story, five of the bridesmaids were lazy procrastinators; five wisely remained prepared even during the prolonged wait for the bridegroom (symbolic of the Lord). The five wise ones were there to meet the bridegroom when he arrived. The others were shut out of the wedding banquet.

I want to be among the wise who will awake each morning with a readiness and gladness of heart to love and serve the Lord and his people, care for his creation and try to bring justice and peace to my world, and, if possible, the larger world. I want my family and friends to know they are God's great gift to me.

I wondered where this knowledge would lead me. I do know that my faith has increased exponentially. My knowledge of God has expanded and deepened. I've been able to comprehend more fully the breadth and length and height and depth of God's power and love.

## FOURTH TREATMENT

I had a CT scan two days before my scheduled fourth treatment. On the day of my treatment I got the scan results from Dr. Meshad. His previous prediction was proven correct. I had multiple tumors throughout my body. The scan showed that all of the tumors had decreased in size by at least 50 percent. Dr. Meshad pronounced me in partial remission. He would discontinue the chemotherapy but would continue with Rituxan, the maintenance drug. My Rituxan treatments would be administered once every two months intravenously until I was in full remission. Because Rituxan is a slow-acting drug it might be two years until my remission was complete. The best news is that Rituxan has few or no side effects. In my case, I had no side effects and could begin to build my strength and return to a more normal life.

I was elated! The prediction Dr. Meshad gave me at our first meeting was that I would be in partial remission between four and six chemotherapy treatments. Instead I had reached that point after three treatments (and most likely after two). Six months later a PET scan indicated that I was in full remission, again much sooner than predicted. Still, I would continue with the maintenance drug every two months.

I know there are many factors that contributed to my quick progress toward remission. Besides the help from my very good medical team and support from family and friends, I also had incorporated some complementary therapies for which I am trained and have used. I believe that prayer and guidance from God have also been major factors in my healing.

These are all described in the following chapters.

# { 3 }

# GOD SPEAKS TO US
# IN MANY WAYS

THERE IS COMMON ACCEPTANCE AMONG Judeo-Christians that God speaks through the word (i.e, the biblical Scriptures, the homilies of clergy, and listening prayer). There seems to be less acknowledgment that God speaks through other vessels. This is a human limitation, though, imposed on us by our narrow thinking processes. Since this planet we live on is God's creation, God has at his disposal the entire creation for communicating with us, for being in relationship with us. God knows that if we don't respond to one language, we may understand and respond to another language—the language of visual art, or music, or poetry, or nature, an innocent comment by a friend or stranger, or through metaphor, symbols, or humor.

The story of Moses' call to rescue the Israelites from their Egyptian oppressor demonstrates God's great sense of humor. Moses, minding his own business one day, led his sheep beyond the wilderness to the mount of Horeb, presumably to better pastures. Along the way he saw a burning bush. A burning bush is not an unusual sight, but this bush continued to burn without being consumed. Moses, being a curious guy, moved closer to see what was going on. From the bush God spoke through an angel, commanding Moses to go to Egypt and lead God's people out of the country. How Moses resisted! He didn't know how to do that. He wasn't a leader. He would have to leave his familiar home and way of life to rescue some folks he had never seen before.

Despite Moses' resistance, God won. For the next forty-plus years Moses led a mass of whining, complaining, disrespectful, disobedient people until they finally found a home in Canaan. All because of a perplexing, unquenchable fire in a bush. Moses must have often wanted to kick himself in the seat of the pants for being so curious. Still, if he hadn't fallen for the burning bush trick, God would have found another way to speak to him. God doesn't give up.

Throughout the Bible, dreams play a significant role in transmitting messages from God. There was a general belief among Hebrew people that dreams were vehicles of divine revelation. They were sometimes conveyed directly and unambiguously. At other times dreams were conveyed through symbolic language, as in the Joseph stories in Genesis, chapters forty and forty-one. Joseph's ability to interpret accurately the symbolism of cows and ears of grain in the dreams of Pharoah earned his release from prison and a promotion to overseer of all the land of Egypt.

The story of Jesus might have been very different if his father, Joseph, hadn't received a direct warning from God in a dream, heeded it, and fled to safety in Egypt with his infant son and Mary. Later, God's instructions as to when and how Joseph could safely return home came to Joseph directly through a dream.

Unfortunately, dreams are no longer thought of as important vehicles for God's messages. Many dismiss dreams as frivolous topics of conversation. Dreams today, however, come from the same source as they did in ancient times—a deep level of consciousness that isn't usually available to us until our mental guards are asleep. Dreams are still prophetic, still great teachers when we give them the attention they deserve.

Music has guided me through many difficult situations in my personal life. When listening to great music there is a sense of knowing beyond knowing. A physician once told me, "When I listen to Brahms I just *know.*" As a music psychotherapist guiding a client through a music-listening experience, I have often heard such responses as "The (solo) trumpet tells me what I must do." Or a dialogue between two solo instruments may initiate an inner dialogue that brings insight into a difficult relationship or some other problematic situation.

There is biblical authority for using music to receive guidance. In the Hebrew Bible there is evidence that during the era of the kings there were guilds of prophets who used music to induce trance states in which they could hear God's messages. In 2 Kings: 3 we read the story of the kings of Israel, Edom, and Judah forming a coalition to fight against an attack by the king of Moab. In assessing their defenses the kings realized there was no water for their army or the animals that supported the army. In great distress they searched for a prophet of God to tell them what to do. The prophet Elisha was summoned. As soon as Elisha heard what they needed he replied, "Get me a musician." The story continues: "And then, while the musician was playing, the power of the Lord came on him." And he prophesied. Elisha's prophecy was good news to the kings, and it was accurate. What occurred was true to what Elisha had prophesied.

Music affects brain waves and alters our consciousness so that the voices of musical instruments can become the voice of God speaking through the instruments.

Often when actively listening to music I have received much-needed insights.

Who has not gazed upon a work of art and been mesmerized by a sense that something has changed within? Great art often communicates something to the viewer that the artist was not aware of when creating it. The artist becomes a vessel for the message intended for the viewer. There is some organic process that causes a shift in the viewer's mental and emotional states and brings a sense of *knowing* that wasn't there before. God is speaking to us through our imagination when we are inspired by shapes and colors that initiate new thoughts or new perspectives on old thoughts.

Nature is alive with revelations of God's glory. The psalmist recognized that God is revealed by the natural world, without benefit of words. In the Old Testament, particularly in Isaiah and the Psalms, nature sings praises to its creator noisily, with spirit and joy. In today's world we can hear nature groaning and howling in pain as it is being systematically destroyed. Yet as I watched a spectacular sunset over Mobile Bay with my son, I realized the earth is still trying to forgive us. Even with its violent treatment by human hands the natural world still gives us soul-healing beauty. That can be explained only by God's love for his creation. The voice of the natural world is so powerful it is heard throughout all the earth.

My unchurched years, the years in which I was rebelling against the church as an institution, were the years in which I had close encounters with God through nature. I spent many weekends hiking and camping in the southern Appalachian mountains in north Georgia, or canoeing through the pristine waters of rivers that could only be accessed by canoe, kayak, or raft. Drinking in, or sometimes gulping, the primeval beauty of those areas, I knew that only God could be the giver of such gifts. God spoke through the sounds of his creation—water rushing over rock, the clattering rattle of a belted kingfisher, the trill of a red-winged blackbird, or the human creation of a crackling fire built at river's edge. I absorbed the ancient wisdom of the silent Appalachians, the oldest mountain range on the planet. I felt the holiness of God's creation all about me. God spoke peace to me. God reshaped and reordered my thoughts, God taught me to be still and silent.

With all of these resources available to me, why would God choose cancer as a transmitter of messages I had not received before? I was adept at hearing and receiving God's truth in so many familiar and pleasing ways. Why now, when I'm in late life, would God choose a way of transmission that would require me to learn a new language— a language of pain, nausea, discomfort, helplessness, and disruption of my normal lifestyle? What could be conveyed through this new language that couldn't have been communicated in the old and familiar ways?

I believe God is in everything, including cancer, but I had never *experienced* God in this kind of bodily invasion. I believe God speaks to us through suffering, but I had never *experienced* God's voice in this way. Perhaps this new experience would reveal something more that God wants me to know.

Father Thack commented in one of his homilies, "There are some things that you can't know or learn from a book, even the Bible. There are some things you have to experience for yourself." He referred to smug, self-satisfied religiosity as "spiritual cataracts" obscuring our vision of God. "Christianity is not, and never has been, about finding the right combination of words," he continued. "It is about encountering the living and loving God, experiencing his presence in the ordinary as well as in the miraculous."

My cancer journey was to be an encounter beyond words.

## FAMILIAR WAYS, NEW EXPERIENCE

I found that some of the familiar means of receiving messages from God could be applied to this new experience of disease. An often tried and very revealing way to find thoughts, feelings, and meanings from the depths of our consciousness is to engage with the problem in a written dialogue. This is not an intellectual dialogue. To be successful you need to push your intellect to the outer fringes of attention and surrender to the intuitive functions of your brain. For example, when dialoguing with cancer it is helpful to personify the cancer. Let the cancer, not your intellect, speak for itself.

Write your dialogue with no attention to grammar or spelling. Simply let it flow in a stream-of-consciousness style. In this way, you're dipping into a deeper level of consciousness, a level that reveals unrecognized or unacknowledged feelings and thoughts. By bringing parts of yourself that have been lying hidden into your awareness you can attend to them. Sometimes you may be surprised by your real feelings. Nevertheless they're there, as if on a large screen. When bringing them to conscious attention, you can eliminate obstacles you hadn't recognized earlier.

To be able to do this kind of dialogue, you must be in a quiet place with no distractions or intrusions. With writing paper and pen in hand, sit in a comfortable position, close your eyes, and focus your attention on your breathing. If thoughts begin interrupting, turn your attention back to your breathing. Concentrate on making your breathing deeper and slower. Do this until the outer world is on the periphery of your awareness, and your attention is on the inner self. This may take some time for those inexperienced in meditation or relaxation techniques, but it's a very helpful practice for many needs in life. I urge you to continue this practice until it becomes natural and easy. The relaxation techniques explained in Appendix B may be useful.

When you've silenced the mental chatter from the outer world and your focus is on your interior world, begin your dialogue. Continue until the dialogue feels completed, i.e., until your cancer has had its say and you've had yours.

Soon after my diagnosis I had a dialogue with my cancer. Here's how it went:

*R(Ruth): What is this thing you're doing to me? Filling my body with poison, tearing down my defenses and my strength, interrupting my life, providing obstacles to everything I've been doing? Why would you do this to me? Have I not tried to live a healthy life, to take care of my body and live a Christian life? What do you want from me?*

*C(Cancer): This is a test—a big one for you.*

*R: Here I am in late life. Haven't I been tested enough? How many tests do I have to go through? And what kind of test is this? What do I get if I pass it? Or fail it?*

*C: More and more about this test will be revealed with time. You can't know this all at once. But who do you think you are that you should not be vulnerable to disease, to things that happen to other people? I am evil incarnate. I take over your body; I test your ability to overcome, to endure, to triumph. I can destroy you. Now, call on your God. We'll see who is the master here.*

*R: My God has power over all evil. He is omnipotent and omnipresent. He is present in this cancer. My faith is in God and his purpose for me.*

Soon after this dialogue occurred I read this Scripture:

*My brothers and sisters, whenever you face trials of any kind, consider it nothing but joy, because you know that the testing of your faith produces endurance; and let endurance have its full effect, so that you may be mature and complete, lacking in nothing (James 1:2-4).*

I prayed:

*Lord, it's so hard to consider cancer as a joy, but I do want to mature in my faith. I open myself to your holiness in every part of my body, mind, and soul. God, the Father, the Son, and the Holy Spirit, enfold me in your grace and love.*

## LECTIO DIVINA

How could I adapt to this new means of communication to receive messages through my cancer? With a willingness to be open I began to find new meaning in the Scriptures and other readings. I began to "hear" many things directly relevant to my illness. I perceived differently. One of the significant ways in which I received messages was through the practice of *lectio divina*.

In her book *Too Deep For Words: Rediscovering Lectio Divina*, Sister Thelma Hall describes *lectio divina* beautifully when she says it is "a holistic way of prayer which disposes, opens and 'informs' us for the gift of contemplation God waits to give, by leading us to a meeting place with him in our deepest center, his life-giving dwelling place." Although this practice dates back to before the sixth century, many of today's Christians know nothing of its existence.

*Lectio divina* is a simple way of praying through the Scriptures and is available to anyone. Sister Hall describes it as a way of "seeing" God, of touching and being touched by him, of "experiencing him." She reminds us that God in himself is another language that speaks to us.

I think one of the reasons *lectio divina* is no longer in common use is because it requires time, patience, and silence. These are unfamiliar gifts and difficult to access in today's busy, noisy world. *Lectio divina* can mean a radical change not only in how we pray, but also in how we live. It leads to an inner awakening to God, to communion with God on a deep, quiet level.

When I read Sister Hall's instructions on how to go about the practice of *lectio divina* I was struck by how much it is like my practice of contemplative prayer. The way I practice it evolved intuitively from a need and desire to encounter God in a deeply personal way. Probably my years of practicing meditation helped me focus in the intense way required in contemplative prayer.

Basically, it begins with *intent*. Intent requires a daily practice, a practice of setting aside an indeterminate time, when possible; of finding a quiet, undisturbed place, and quietening your mind. The breathing exercises in Appendix B may help you learn to calm your mind and move your focus from the external world to the interior. The preparation stage also involves asking God to be in your experience, to speak to you and let you know whatever he wants you to know at that time.

This is followed by *reading* the Scriptures. I use the daily Scriptures suggested in the lectionary of the Book of Common Prayer in the Episcopal Church. Sometimes I use additional Scriptures that I'm drawn to on any given day, or a commentary from *Forward Day by Day*. If you're a member of another church and don't have access to the Book of Common Prayer, you might ask a minister or spiritual director to suggest Scriptures appropriate for your need.

Reading is followed by *meditation* on the Scriptures—a reflection on the meaning of what you have just read. Meditation primarily engages the intellect, however. When you wait patiently, meditation may bring you closer to an intimate inner dialogue with God. Your experience may then transition to what some refer to as a "prayer of the heart." As the heart takes over, there is often an outpouring of love and desire for God.

When praying through the Scriptures in the early stages of my illness I felt a deep need to regain my equilibrium, to understand, to get wise advice. My needs drew me into the Scriptures like a magnet, carrying me far beyond the words on a printed page to the power generated by them. Moving through and being moved by the Scriptures, I felt myself caught up in God's astonishing wisdom. The Scriptures came alive and made themselves fully present to me.

When we are praying the prayer of the heart we are beginning to enter the state of consciousness that Sister Hall refers to as "too deep for words." It is a state in which all mental chatter is silenced, a state of being in which we can patiently wait for God. This is the prayer in which we can become immersed in God. We may "hear" God speak, or we may simply rest in God's presence.

Theologian Henri Nouwen speaks of the profound nature of the prayer of the heart. He states that when we pray the prayer of the heart "all those who have become part of our lives are led into the healing presence of God and touched by him in the center of our being." Because God's heart has become one with ours, our hearts can embrace "all human pain and sorrow, all conflicts and agonies, all torture and war, all hunger, loneliness, and misery." It's difficult to fully comprehend this amazing ability of the open heart to be a first responder, to enfold all human troubles and offer itself as the center of connection with the healing God.

Theologically, contemplative prayer is based on Jesus' instructions in Matthew 6:6:

> *But whenever you pray, go into your room and shut the*
> *door and pray to your Father in secret; and your Father*
> *who sees in secret will reward you.*

Irish Jesuit priest William Johnston speaks of contemplative prayer as being "vertical meditation," because it "spirals down into its own silent depths, to the core of the being." This kind of prayer goes beyond rational thinking processes, *involving the whole person* in both rational and intuitive capabilities.

The state of inner stillness, with mental chatter silenced, is the point at which we can access the "Spirit of Truth, the Holy Spirit, the Advocate" promised by Saint John in his gospel.

> *But the Advocate, the Holy Spirit, whom the Father will*
> *send in my name, will teach you everything, and remind*
> *you of all that I have said to you* (John 14:26).

In contemplative prayer sometimes you may receive words or thoughts that are simply implanted in your mind. I find it useful to write these in my journal when the prayer is over. It's important, though, not to get anxious or think you're not doing it right when there is only silence during the prayer. At times silence is God's language. Resting in God's silence is its own reward.

# { 4 }

# IN THE CRUCIBLE

A S MY CHEMOTHERAPY TREATMENTS PROGRESSED with debilitating effects, I began to think of cancer as a crucible. A crucible is a container used for calcining metals and ores with intense heat. What comes out of the crucible is different from what went in. "Crucible" may also be defined as a test or difficult trial.

On my sickest days I thought of my illness as a crucible of faith. What was being poured into the crucible were my strengths and weaknesses, faults and virtues, faith and doubt. All the substances of my being were emptied into the white heat to be reshaped. What shape would emerge from the crucible? I hoped this flawed me would be re-formed into a person more pleasing to God.

The invisible is as much a part of our reality as the visible. This disease was invisible while it gained strength. Not only were there no outer symptoms, but it wasn't even visible to medical tests until it had reached an advanced stage. I pondered: If this insidious cancer is a metaphor for some part of my life invisible to me, or unrecognized by me, what is it? I read: ". . . God, through Jesus Christ, will judge the secret thoughts of all" (Romans 2:16).

Petty, cynical thoughts arising spontaneously are not worthy of Christ. As conscientious Christians we need to be aware of such unspoken thoughts. They aren't secret to God, and *neither are they secret to our bodies.* Unchecked, they accumulate in the confines of the body. Just as swollen lymph glands can block the healthy functioning of our internal organs, so can unchristian thoughts block the healthy flow of Christian living. In such an environment the living Christ lacks an unfettered space within which to guide us. How can Christ's spirit coexist in a mind and body full of unholy thoughts?

I read in Paul's letter to the Ephesians: ". . . but everything exposed by the light becomes visible . . ." (5:13).

CT and PET scans expose what is inside the body, hidden from our view. Would that our obstructions to God's will be exposed as easily. One of my obstacles has been a resistance to a complete surrender to trusting in God. Trusting that God in his infinite wisdom will carry those I love safely through difficult times, give them the discernment they need, and guide them in wise decision-making means letting go of my interference, no matter how many times I have to swallow my words.

I sometimes let petty annoyances get in the way of being immersed in God. I let the trivial, superficial life of the world keep me from living the true reality—the reality that we live, move, and have our being in God. Believing—and living otherwise—is to deny the ultimate power of God, through whom all things are possible.

In Paul's first letter to the Thessalonians he reminds us: ". . . you are all children of light and children of the day . . ." (5:5).

I think Paul is telling us to live as if there's a great light shining on us, revealing our actions, even the state of our thoughts and the nature of our hearts. Such a light would surely keep us vigilant, so as not to be shamed by an inner nature that can safely hide in the darkness. It might enable us to show love and mercy even in our secret thoughts.

One morning I read: "This illness does not lead to death; rather it is for God's glory, so that the Son of God may be glorified through it" (John 11:4). I didn't know if cancer would lead to my death. Still, I wondered if there was a way my illness might reflect God's glory?

Other Scriptures spoke to me: ". . . for he is like a refiner's fire . . . and he will refine them like gold and silver until they present offerings to the Lord in righteousness" (Malachi 3:2b-3).

I wondered what offerings I needed to present. The author of Hebrews spoke to me: "Because he himself was tested by what he suffered, he is able to help those who are being tested" (2:18).

What I have learned from the challenges of this illness may be of help to others facing similar tests. I can offer that help to anyone who wants it. I prayed the prayer of the psalmist:

> *O God, from my youth you have taught me and I still proclaim your wondrous deeds. So even to old age and gray hairs, O God, do not forsake me until I proclaim your might to all the generations to come. Your power and your righteousness, O God, reach the high heavens* (Psalms 71:17-18).

An offering would be to proclaim the power and wonder of God that is revealed to me through this illness. God had led me to untried experiences. I could reveal what I have learned from them.

39

How could I make these offerings? A book came to mind when I began to receive God's messages of guidance. A book is a major project, however, involving many days, weeks and months of work, and enormous creative energy. How could I explain this experience in a way that would make a difference to people facing similar tests? The answer came: "Do not worry about . . . what to say, because when the time comes, the Holy Spirit will teach you what you should say" (Luke 12:11-12).

That passage gave me the courage to begin writing this book. I was reassured, in believing that I would not be alone in doing it.

## DEALING WITH THE STIGMA

There is now much more knowledge about cancer than in previous years and a wider realization that it happens often among our families and friends. That knowledge has resulted in cancer becoming more normalized in our world. Yet there is still some stigma attached to it. I had a sense of some people backing off when they learned I had cancer, even though physically they hadn't moved an inch. I began to realize that some people deep in their hearts worry that cancer is contagious, although intellectually they know it isn't. Or perhaps their fear of the disease itself created more distance.

I was concerned that there might be some parishioners at St. Paul's who would be fearful of my drinking from the common cup during the Eucharist. I began to dip the wafer into the wine rather than drinking from the cup.

One day I received a call from a woman who wanted to take piano lessons. I was in the throes of the debilitating effects of chemotherapy, and I knew I couldn't take her as a student until I was feeling better. I explained to her that I would be glad to accept her as a student when I was finished with the chemotherapy treatments. I offered to let her know when that time came. She immediately began to back off and make excuses for not beginning lessons. Eventually, she revealed that her mother had died of cancer and she just couldn't follow through with lessons from me. After apologizing, she hung up. When reflecting on her behavior I realized she was probably still grieving her mother's death and was fearful of developing a relationship with anyone who had the same disease that had killed her mother.

I wanted to be sensitive to the fears of others, yet I refused to be defined by cancer. In my years of practice in psychotherapy I sometimes worked with clients who were diagnosed with cancer. They often expressed the sadness that their former identity was changed by the diagnosis. They were no longer identified as a teacher, a successful businessperson, or a musician. They were now identified as a cancer patient by their medical team as well as by friends and coworkers. I refused that identity change. I was still me, only with the addition of having cancer.

## AT THE HAND OF THE PRUNER

During chemotherapy treatments, some of the activities that had sustained me during difficult times in the past became unavailable: singing, journaling, gardening, and playing the piano.

Singing restores energy and changes moods as sound waves move through the body. The vibratory energy initiated when singing or simply making nonsensical sounds with the voice allows for the expression of any emotion.

Voice movement therapist Paul Newham explains that sounds produced by an individual provide an intimate touching within the body. Singing is like an inward stroking, a gentle stimulation of the muscles, bones, cells, organs, and tissues. Because sounds are vibrations, singing affects the involuntary functions of the body—the heart rate, breathing rate, and circulation; the nervous, endocrine, and digestive systems—in a positive way. Singing also brings a person to a sense of self. The singer produces the tones, can change them in any way, direct them to any part of the body, and experience the strong, kinesthetic sensations of sound waves moving through the body. Singing reduces the sense of alienation with self by offering intimate connection. Our body as an acoustic vessel reverberates when sound is initiated. Those internal reverberations provide a kinesthetic image of us much as a mirror reflects a self-image visually.

In the judgment of Newham, "Singing gives dominion to those without territory, passes time for those who await judgment, and gives voice to a part of the soul which cannot be beaten, broken or beleaguered."

Singing in the choir each Sunday had been, for me, a particularly grace-filled form of worship. The cancer damaged a nerve to my vocal chords, and my voice became squeaky, high-pitched, and weak. Singing was no longer possible. Even on days when I felt like singing, my voice let me down. Even if God "put a new song in my mouth" (Psalms 40:3) as he did for the psalmist, I couldn't express it audibly. I would have to find some other way to worship.

Playing the piano has always focused my mind and spirit on the beauty of the classics. It allows me to shut out all distractions and enter my internal world. It centers me in times of chaos and restores serenity. But my hands became shaky and weak as a result of the chemotherapy. During times when playing would have been a normal way to uplift myself, trying to play now became a frustrating chore.

Gardening has long been a spiritual practice for me. When I moved into my present house my goal was to make of my house and yard a sanctuary for friends, family, butterflies, birds—and me. Planting, digging in the soil, and nurturing what I plant immerses me in the intimacy of caring for God's creation.

On the eastern shore of Mobile Bay we are on the pathway of one of the most important migration routes of many diverse birds going from north to south and south to north. For those migrating birds and for the many that remain in our area year-round, I had kept food and water available. With the cancer I became physically unable to garden, or even to replenish the bird feeder. When my longtime friend and fellow bird lover Diane spent a week with me after the second treatment, she carefully cleaned out the feeder and kept it filled with seeds. The birds joyfully thanked us by showing up with their beautiful colors.

Journaling in the form of free-flowing writing without regard to grammar, spelling, and syntax had been a significant way to put down spontaneous thoughts and feelings without judgment. This practice provides rich material for later reflection and meditation. It can also be the source of internal dialogue and a tool to discover unrecognized obstacles to leading a healthy and spiritual life. There were many days following chemotherapy treatments that I was simply too sick or tired to journal. When I read a passage in the Gospel of John I felt the evangelist was speaking directly to me: "Every branch that bears fruit, he prunes to make it bear more fruit" (14:2).

God was pruning me, cutting off the familiar sustaining resources so that I would be forced to search elsewhere for aid, comfort, and meaning. Without the familiar and comfortable aids, my sustenance was to be narrowed and refined so that I would listen more deeply to what God wanted me to hear. God lopped off my branches. Where would the new growth appear? What would the new fruits look like?

While lying in bed I discovered *internal journaling* to be a way of bearing much fruit. Lying in bed became boring, yet I was too sick to get up and do anything. In the silent waiting, thoughts, insights, and messages emerged in a free-flowing pattern. It was like having a casual conversation with a friend. Among friends the dialogue often wanders comfortably, with no known agenda, until eventually it becomes clear what the real conversation is all about.

The ponderings and wanderings in our silent time leave us open and unguarded so that God can narrow our focus and gently lead our thoughts, eventually homing in on what God wants us to see and hear. In the silence of my suffering, thoughts and internal dialogues were being written and sealed on my heart. At a later time, when I felt stronger, my heart would release those thoughts so I could write them on the pages of my journal.

Later, in my *lectio divina* time I read in Jeremiah 31:33b: "I will put my law within them, and I will write it on their hearts, and I will be their God and they shall be my people."

God is such an opportunist! He brought me to my knees, helpless in my sickness, and he seized the moment to silently implant his wisdom in my mind and heart.

*Though the Lord may give you the bread of adversity
and the water of affliction, yet your Teacher will not
hide himself any more, but your eyes shall see your
Teacher. And when you turn to the right or when you
turn to the left, your ears shall hear a word behind you,
saying, "This is the way; walk in it"* (Isaiah 30:20-21).

This was a covenant between God and me. God would always
be present, guiding me every day, every moment, with every breath.
There would be no excuses for not walking in God's way. I, in turn,
would be committed to walking the way.


## A New Spirit

My Scripture reading one morning was Ezekiel 36:26-27: "A
new heart I will give you . . . I will put my spirit within you."

I prayed:

*Lord, put your spirit within me—the spirit with so much
love and faith that I will follow you anywhere.*

I have always asked for the faith that would move mountains. I
pondered: Is this whole cancer thing about deepening my faith? The
apostle Paul thought that walking the walk of faith was following
God into the unknown, risky, and challenging regions where God
dwells, trusting that God is in charge. Cancer has certainly taken
me into the unknown. Every treatment is a new and challenging
experience—difficult and unpleasant, relying a lot on the help of
other people, something I haven't been accustomed to doing. It

has also given other people the opportunity to offer themselves to help me get through this. I wondered: Is this for the sake of other people too?

Something rises within us—the better part of ourselves—when we're given the opportunity to help someone, not because we should, but simply because we want to. There's something about being a Good Samaritan that connects us with the reality of what being a disciple means, that allows us to experience the joy in obeying Jesus' instructions to care for others. I think of the many folks who have so warmly and graciously helped me. Had my cancer and neediness somehow been a blessing for them?

When my friend Emily read the above paragraphs her answer was, "Yes, it has been a blessing." She pointed out that when family members or friends are really sick or injured, we have a feeling of helplessness. It hurts to see them suffering, and we know we can't make them well. She adds, "When our help is offered and accepted, we no longer feel completely hopeless and helpless."

In Mark 8 Jesus reminded his disciples of the occasion when he had fed five thousand people with five loaves of bread, and on another occasion four thousand people with seven loaves. "Do you not yet understand?" he asked (21).

In giving, the gift is multiplied many times over. In serving others, the service is increased in many ways that can't readily be seen. We give and serve because we are God's beloved children. The manifestation of our giving and serving can be profound and astonishing, in the same way that a butterfly flitting over my garden in Daphne can cause events to occur in a faraway place. It occurs to me that evil can have the same universal effect, so we must concentrate on the good to neutralize evil.

*So we do not lose heart. Even though our outer nature is wasting away, our inner nature is being renewed day by day. For this light momentary affliction is preparing us for an eternal weight of glory beyond all measure, because we look not at what can be seen but at what cannot be seen; for what can be seen is temporary, but what cannot be seen is eternal* (2 Corinthians 4:16-18).

Our most authentic nature is at the soul level, the level at which we meet the Christ within, the level that cannot be seen from the outside. When Jesus said, "Do not judge by appearances, but judge with right judgment" (John 7:24), he is instructing us to look at the Christ within every person. This can be very difficult when a person's views—political, social, spiritual, and philosophical—conflict with ours. But when we can go beyond outer appearances and connect with that person at the soul level, the truth—the right judgment—will reveal itself. The unseen may be where the deeper truth lies.

# { 5 }

# INTEGRATIVE MEDICINE

I NTEGRATIVE MEDICINE (IM) IS A newly emerging field that has evolved from complementary and alternative medicine (CAM). CAM is a multibillion dollar, unregulated industry with potential benefits and risks to consumers, including cancer patients. For many years the medical field didn't recognize alternative therapies, and with good reason. Alternative therapies were used to *replace* conventional medicine, and some involved risky practices. They were untested, unregulated, and often used by "practitioners" who had no credible training.

Complementary therapies, however, are used *together* with conventional medicine. In recent years some CAM therapies have gained credibility because of research proving scientifically that they augment conventional medicine. Thus, many doctors are now embracing integrative medicine that incorporates safe and effective complementary therapies. The acceptance by physicians of these additions to conventional medicine helps to ensure that patients are treated as whole persons.

Psychologist Larry LeShan spent many years in research with terminally ill cancer patients, trying to find what he calls a "mobilizing life force," the self-healing capacity within the human body that would allow his patients not only to survive but also to thrive. In an interview he commented, "What patients can do is set an example for the immune system by treating themselves as if they are really worth caring for, as if they are special, as if their life is worth fighting for." This suggests a strong effect from a positive dialogue between patient and immune system.

When patients are permitted to choose the complementary therapies that most appeal to them, they become part of a team effort in their treatment plan. The combination of therapies, medicine, and active patient participation becomes what is known as holistic medicine. Among the therapies that are now recognized and gradually becoming mainstream in cancer care are music therapy, imagery, expressive writing, and relaxation techniques. Some of the large comprehensive cancer centers in the United States and other countries have integrated these and other therapies and have on their staffs professionally trained therapists in these fields.

Music, imagery (music-initiated imagery in particular), relaxation, and expressive writing are therapies in which I have been trained, have practiced extensively, and taught to other therapists. Since I know firsthand how effective they are in the healing process I added them to my own treatment.

I was once talking to a man about the healing benefits of music. He responded quite sharply by saying that healing occurs only through Jesus Christ. Of course Jesus is the source, but God works his works through all of his creation. When we try to keep God's works contained within the perceptions of our own limited minds we make God small. The God I know heals through doctors, antibiotics, and mental health counselors. God heals through the beauty of nature, through a kind word, through the Scriptures and prayer. And God heals through music, his great gift to us. Why else would that creation be available to us? How else could all the sounds within the universe be heard, organized, and transformed by gifted musicians into music that calms the mind and stirs the soul? Unfortunately, there is sound in our world that is neither calming nor soul-stirring. In choosing music for healing we need to be discerning.

In addition to using these complementary therapies I integrated prayer with my medical treatments. I didn't set out to make a treatment plan. These are just things I have practiced for many years. They transferred quite naturally into my life with cancer. Anyone who wants to can incorporate these activities into his or her own treatment. They are safe, noninvasive, inexpensive, and beneficial. The following descriptions may be of help to those who want to use them in their own healing. Prayer is discussed separately in Chapter 6.

## MUSIC

Music's ability to bring beauty to our lives and transform moods quickly is universally known and accepted. The power of music to heal is less understood. Its ability to make a significant contribution to the treatment of many illnesses isn't sufficiently recognized and, therefore, is underused. Music as a surrogate support group is one such example.

Some studies have demonstrated that cancer patients who are in support groups experience an improvement in quality of life and, in some cases, extended survival times.

Patients in cancer support groups express a better sense of control over their lives and decreased feelings of isolation when they are among others who *understand* the difficulties they're experiencing. Hearing others express similar feelings of anxiety, fears, frustration, and their very real difficulties in living with decreased physical capacity helps patients to be less lonely. They feel they are understood. They have others with whom they can talk with honesty about their difficulties. Some may feel they need to protect family members and cannot speak to them openly about their cancer. For patients in a support group the improved quality of life may very well improve the quality of dying for those who don't survive the cancer.

Although there are now internet support groups, many patients don't have access to a support group. Others choose not to be part of a group. For those patients, music can provide much-needed psychological and emotional support. For patients who are in a support group, music can enhance the psychological benefits gained from the group.

Music can be most supportive when it's chosen according to the isomorphic principle (i.e., matching music to mood). When a person is feeling tense and anxious, a choice of "happy" music is counterproductive. The psychological dissonance between the person's feelings and the mood of the music creates more tension. It's as if the "happy" music is saying to the person, "No, no, your feelings aren't valid. You shouldn't feel that way."

Choosing music that matches tense, anxious feelings validates the individual's feelings. It is music that *understands* and *supports*. It lends the necessary support for persons to move *through* their feelings rather than *around* them. Music can aid in the expression of feelings that can't be expressed in words. After moving through anxiety and other feelings, the sense of relief is cathartic. It brings a sense of accomplishment to the individual and reduces the feeling of helplessness in a situation where there is so little control over what happens. On a spiritual level, going deeply into the experience of anxiety, pain, helplessness, and other feelings—rather than bypassing them—attunes us to universal suffering. Our perceptions change as we realize there are no strangers in suffering. We are the "one body" that we Christians proclaim.

When preparing for my first chemotherapy treatment I selected several music programs to take with me. These were programs that I had compiled for therapeutic use with clients in my psychotherapy practice. A list of the music I chose can be found in Appendix D.

Since I am a classically trained pianist, my preference is music of a classical nature. However, I have found that this music also often helps people whose first choice of music is something other than classical. If your preference is for other music styles I suggest that you take some time before your cancer treatments to select music you feel will support and comfort you. One thing to keep in mind is that music chosen for recreational listening may not meet the criteria of providing comfort and alleviating anxiety in very stressful situations.

The power of music to heal has been known since ancient times. In 1 Samuel 16:14-23 we read how the young David cured King Saul of his psychotic episodes by playing on his lyre. "Now the spirit of the Lord departed from Saul, and an evil spirit from the Lord tormented him." Saul's servants suggested to the king that he find someone skilled at playing the lyre, "and when the evil spirit from God is upon you, he will play it, and you will feel better." King Saul listened and put out a search for a musician. David, a young shepherd and skilled lyre musician, was found and brought to King Saul. "And whenever the evil spirit from God came upon Saul, David took the lyre and played it with his hand, and Saul would be relieved and feel better, and the evil spirit would depart from him."

It was widely believed in those ancient times that musicians—and by extension music—would ward off evil spirits (mental illness in today's language). People who work in the field of music therapy today know that the belief is factual and just as true today as it was then. A good choice of music can restore order to the chaotic thoughts initiated by a diagnosis of cancer or any other disturbing events.

There is more to music in healing, though. Studies on music and the immune system have shown that music alone has independent influences on the immune system, specifically in the recovery of normal white blood cell activity. The immune system works through the production of white blood cells. The cells have receptors that adversely affect the immune system during extended periods of stress. During prolonged stress the adrenal glands are secreting higher than normal levels of cortisol, a stress hormone. Cortisol belongs to a group of steroids called glucocorticoids, which are known to decrease the potency of the immune response. When calming music reaches the brain through the auditory cortex, glucocorticoid production is decreased. The result is improved recovery of normal white blood cell activity.

Following my second chemotherapy treatment, Dr. Meshad omitted the injection of Neulaste, which is designed to help in recovery of white blood cells. In spite of the omission of Neulaste, the bloodwork just prior to the third treatment showed that my white blood cell count was "good" (Dr. Meshad's assessment).

I cannot prove that the recovery of my white blood cell count without an injection of Neulaste was enhanced by my use of music. However, as soon as each treatment began, I started listening to the music I had compiled and brought with me. It seems reasonable to hypothesize: Along with the infusion of chemotherapy drugs that *decrease* the number of white blood cells, the musical sound waves entering my body were positively influencing the functioning of my immune system, assisting in the *increase* of white blood cells.

I know that listening to music reduced the stress I felt at the beginning of treatment and kept me calm throughout. Music also helped to reduce the adverse effects of the throbbing aches in my body in the first two weeks following each treatment. The fascinating act of *entrainment* occurs when rhythms within our body (e.g., breathing and heart rate) begin to match the rhythms and tempo of music. When listening to music with a tempo of somewhere around 72 beats per minute (the approximate rate of a healthy heart at rest), our breathing and heart rate adjust to that tempo. Slowing our body rhythms brings a calming effect that helps us to relax, and it reduces feelings of stress. The calming effect alleviates aches and pain. In addition, music aids in the release of endorphins, the body's natural opiate. Music can bring the same kind of high that runners experience by altering brain wave activity. It serves as both a distraction and an anesthetic.

## IMAGERY

Images are electrochemical events in the body. They communicate with tissues, organs, and cells and are capable of initiating profound physiological changes. Psychologist Jeanne

Achterberg describes imagery as "the thought process that invokes and uses the senses: vision, audition, smell, taste, movement, position, and touch. It is the communication mechanism between perception, emotion, and bodily change." The fathers of medicine—the ancient Greeks Asclepius, Aristotle, Galen, and Hippocrates—used imagery for both diagnosis and therapy.

The imagination isn't often recognized as a part of health care. However, every interaction with doctors and other health care practitioners, and every conversation about diagnosis and treatment, creates internal images that strongly affect the course of a disease. The imagery from these interactions impacts the patient either positively or negatively.

Images are also a method of diagnosis, as we know from CT and PET scans and MRIs (magnetic resonance imaging). Images from within the patient's own intuitive brain can also provide diagnoses that are not visible on the medical imaging screens. One of my clients, a man who was diagnosed with an inoperable malignant brain tumor, came for therapy to improve the quality of his remaining life. In our first session I chose music to access a level of consciousness deeper than his ordinary state and to evoke imagery from within him. When he was deeply into his internal world the patient "saw" two tumors—one in profile and one looking straight ahead. A later scan confirmed that he did, indeed, have not one, but two tumors.

Imagery can be used in mental rehearsals as preparation for upcoming chemotherapy or radiation treatment, surgery, or other events that induce anxiety.

Imagery can also be used to enhance healing from cancer or other illnesses. Studies have revealed that the immune system is under direct control of the areas of the brain involved in the transmission of images to the body. Images of healing will have a more beneficial effect on the immune system than images of sickness or death.

Images arising spontaneously from within the person are more engaging than images from a script coming from someone else's imagination. Imagery that may be effective for one person may be irrelevant in the life of another. And, if irrelevant, it won't be as effective as hoped. When imagery arises from within, the imager owns the images. It's as if they're in his DNA because they come from the very fabric of his being. The imagery will then continue to impact his life in ways that can be very helpful.

For example, in one music psychotherapy session I asked a terminally ill client to envision an inner helper. Almost immediately his beloved bird dogs appeared to him, surrounding him, licking his tumors. Never could I have produced imagery that would have been as effective in giving him comfort and support. His dogs continued to be his helpers until his death.

One image I used in my own healing was simply that of divine energy flowing through my body, from head to toe, accessing all parts of my body. That may not be the most beneficial image for someone else. I suggest that you let your images flow as they will, arising from your own life experience.

## MUSIC-EVOKED IMAGERY

Music is one of the most powerful sources for initiating internal imagery. Those who are trained in the Bonny Method of Guided Imagery and Music (BMGIM) know this through observation and practice. BMGIM is a form of depth psychotherapy that uses music-evoked imagery as a vessel for healing and transformation.

Studies have corroborated the effectiveness of music on imagery. Jennie Band, while completing a doctoral degree in counseling education in 1996, explored the effectiveness of music on imagery as compared to imagery experienced in silence or evoked by the verbal suggestions of a guide. Her subjects were college students in a music appreciation class. The music selections she chose for the music-imagery group were J. S. Bach's "Little Fugue" in G minor and Claude Debussy's "En Bateau."

Band's findings were that imagery was much more vigorous and active, colors brighter, and emotions more intense when initiated by music. In addition, memories retrieved in the experiment were more clear, and the degree of absorption in the imagery was substantially increased with the use of music, when compared with imagery experienced in silence or elicited through verbal suggestion.

Thus, when using music to initiate imagery it's essential to use music without words. Music accompanied by lyrics is someone else's script. It will program your imagery based on another person's life experience. If the purpose is to initiate imagery from your deepest self, allowing your own thoughts and feelings to rise to conscious awareness, music without a script (lyrics) is necessary.

Additionally, when using nonverbal music to engage imagery, resistance to words—the everyday, familiar, and sometimes threatening mode of communication—is removed. When images are induced by music rather than by the spoken words of a guide, the risk of imposing someone else's belief system on the listener is significantly reduced. Music is multidimensional and, therefore, much more engaging. It is apt to bring quicker and deeper responses than imagery initiated by the one dimension of spoken language.

For the cancer patient, music-evoked imagery may allow the expression of suppressed feelings, provide images of healing unique to the person, engage attention away from pain and nausea, and give the sense of wonder that comes from accessing our most authentic self. It helps to build trust in inner resources for self-healing.

If you want to experience this method, here's how to do it:

Choose your listening program. It can be something from the lists in Appendix D, or it can be something you have compiled from favorite music or a program on a compact disc that you like. Begin with a focusing, or relaxation, exercise to turn your attention away from the external world. It may help to use one of the breathing exercises in Appendix B.

For those who are inexperienced with focusing techniques I suggest you choose someone to read the exercise aloud while you lie comfortably with your eyes closed. When your attention is sufficiently focused inward, have your helper turn on your selected music. Listen intently, allowing images to emerge freely without trying to analyze them. At the end of the music remain quiet, reflecting on your experience. Journaling or expressive writing at the end may prolong and deepen your experience.

It may also initiate other insights.

## EXPRESSIVE WRITING

Expressive writing, also referred to as journaling, may not be therapeutic for all patients. After a study of patients in a comprehensive cancer treatment center, the authors reported that some patients became upset when writing about their cancer. When I was writing this book one woman I met was amazed that I could write about my cancer. She told me that her cancer had brought such fear she couldn't even talk about it, much less write about it.

As a psychotherapist, however, I found that expressive writing was beneficial to my clients. One man filled three notebooks by keeping a journal in his truck. Every time he stopped for a traffic light he would write the thoughts he had been having as he drove. He said it was like carrying his own therapist in his pocket. Personally, I found expressive writing very helpful in my cancer journey.

Expressive writing is of the greatest benefit when the writer knows that no one will read what is being written, unless by permission. Thus, the fear of judgment is removed. As with any of the expressive arts therapies, when doing expressive writing the intellect should be moved to the sidelines, allowing the intuitive part of the brain freedom to emerge. When thoughts are allowed to flow into words in a stream-of-consciousness style, without attention to grammar, syntax, or spelling, feelings and thoughts not previously recognized or acknowledged can emerge. Repressed feelings can be expressed and emptied. Negative thoughts and feelings can be transferred from within the person to the outside—to the pages of a journal—and left there. It's similar to inducing vomiting to eliminate an intake of poison. The result of a discharge of poisonous thoughts is a feeling of having had a deep cleansing. In the space left clean there is room for healthier thoughts and wiser words to emerge.

We might well look upon expressive writing as guidance from the *inner divine*. Results are often reduced stress and anxiety, better sleeping habits, and helpful—even astonishing—insights.

In my description of *lectio divina* I mentioned that I often received insights from writing in my journal. At times I look back on what I wrote much earlier and am stunned at the new thoughts that spring from the reading. As we evolve and grow we can detect the messages hidden in our earlier writing, waiting to be revealed when we're ready to receive them. Sometimes we innocently bury valuable gems that remain safe until we can recognize their value. This can happen when our attention is focused internally rather than on the outer world.

Unlike listening to music, expressive writing requires some physical energy. There were days when I didn't have the energy to write, or when my hand was too shaky to write. On those days music-listening and imagery, which require less energy, were still available to me.

## THE HEALING BENEFITS OF NATURE

There is a growing recognition that the natural world provides enormous healing benefits for mental and physical health needs. For this reason, I include access to nature as a therapy that complements and enhances conventional medicine. Recent studies have shown strong evidence of the restorative impact of nature on humans—viewing nature and being in nature. People with access to natural settings have been found not only to be healthier than other individuals, but also to have higher levels of satisfaction with life in general.

A study of recovery rates of patients who underwent gall bladder surgery reported that those with a view of a natural setting recovered faster, spent less time in the hospital, required fewer painkillers, and had fewer postoperative complications than patients whose view from the hospital window was of an urban scene. Other studies support these findings. Contact with nature positively impacts blood pressure, cholesterol, outlook on life, and stress-reduction.

Some hospitals have used this knowledge by incorporating patient-centered designs in their buildings. Some have added healing gardens to their facilities. Access to natural areas can be seen as one of our most vital and unrecognized health resources. Certainly, the architects of the Southern Cancer Center were aware of this. It's evident throughout the building and grounds.

Whether in a hospital or at home, cancer patients can improve their environment by opening blinds or curtains to provide more light. Bringing the outside world in expands the perceived boundaries of our life, releasing the sense of physical limitations that accompany cancer. A brief walk outdoors will provide a fresh outlook. If that's not possible, a ride to a park or other natural setting may help. Simply viewing nature has been found to be uplifting. When my friend Diane cleaned and filled the bird feeder, the sight of colorful birds flocking to the feeder brought instant joy to both of us. The beauty of the brilliant, deep blue of indigo buntings and the sharp contrast of the black, white, and red of the red-headed woodpecker always takes my breath away. In those breathless moments pain, fatigue, discomfort, and other concerns are forgotten.

One day Diane brought some flowers in from my garden. That simple act filled a need in both of us for beauty and a reminder that, no matter what, we are part of the natural world. When accessing any part of nature we feel our smallness reaching out to the larger whole that embraces us. Breathing in the wonder of God's natural world instills gratitude within us for its creation and a desire to safeguard "this fragile earth, our island home," as we say in the eucharist liturgy. It is our home, and we're reminded of it when we can focus away from the man-made creations of concrete, asphalt, communication towers, and other such elements of modern genius, and realize the mighty power of God in foreseeing the essential interdependence of all of creation. Home is where God is, and there is no place where God is more at home than in the miracles of nature. When the world was being formed God, in his omnipotence, must surely have planned how healing the natural world would be to his people.

# { 6 }

# RELIGION, SPIRITUALITY, AND PRAYER

**B**ENEDICT CAREY REPORTED IN THE *New York Times* in 2006 that a ten-year scientific investigation of the effectiveness of intercessory prayer on healing had just been completed. The conclusion of the research was that prayers offered by strangers had no effect on the recovery of people undergoing heart surgery. This research, which cost $2.4 million and was led by well-known cardiologist Dr. Herbert Benson, was intended to overcome flaws in earlier investigations on prayer. The results from the latter investigation brought contradictory responses similar to those from previous research.

One response, from Dr. Richard Sloan, professor of behavioral medicine at Columbia University, was, "The problem with studying religion scientifically is that you do violence to the phenomenon by reducing it to basic elements that can be quantified, and that makes for bad science and bad religion." Bob Barth, spiritual director of Silent Unity, a Missouri prayer ministry, responded, "A person of faith would say that this study is interesting, but we've been praying a long time and we've seen prayer work. We know it works and the research on prayer and spirituality is just getting started."

Benson's study included only intercessory prayer from persons unknown to the one being prayed for. It did not include anything about the power of personal prayer or prayers offered by friends and family members.

A 1999 study reported in *Psycho-Oncology* on the role of religion and spirituality in cancer care found significant relationships between religiosity, spirituality, and social dimensions influencing the mental health of patients. Cancer patients described their religious and spiritual beliefs as providing a profound method of coping with the disease and improving their quality of life. Many patients said they relied on spiritual well-being to help them cope with pain, fatigue, and decreased physical ability. Being associated with a church helped to decrease their feelings of isolation and loneliness.

The authors of this study defined religion as "adherence to beliefs, values, and practices proposed by an organized institution devoted to the search for the divine through prescribed ways of viewing and living life." Spirituality was defined as "a search for the sacred or divine through any life experience or route."

Scientific studies notwithstanding, other research has shown that the most common coping strategies for cancer patients was praying alone, praying with others, or having others pray for them. As soon as I was diagnosed with cancer my name was added to the St. Paul's prayer list and prayer lists from other churches. I knew that many people were praying for me every day. I've never been involved in a scientific investigation on the power of prayer. I do know that feeling wrapped in the prayers of so many people fed me, uplifted me, and kept me grounded in the knowledge that Christ is living and very present.

In a lecture for the Oklahoma State LPN Association, Baptist minister Dr. Bruce Prescott commented that science cannot demonstrate that God exists or that God answers prayer. He insists that no one, not even scientists, can put God to the test. "We pray," he says, "because it is an act of worship." He continues, "The act of prayer is an acknowledgment that we depend on power and grace that is beyond ourselves. Nothing demonstrates our dependence on a power that is beyond ourselves more than life-threatening injuries or terminal illness."

Dr. Prescott believes we have gone too far in separating medical science and faith. The growing acknowledgment that mind, body, and spirit are interrelated will bring us to an acceptance of the value of treating the whole person. All of us—patients and medical professionals—will benefit from that approach.

Prayer doesn't have to be confined to a certain time or place or a certain routine. My practice of *lectio divina* usually occurs first thing in the morning when I'm fresh. But contemplative prayer in the morning encourages continuing prayer throughout the day.

Praying is recognizing the presence of God in the moment. I can acknowledge God's presence by praying when I'm working in my garden—watering, weeding, deadheading. I can pray when I'm cleaning the kitchen or cooking a meal. I can pray for patience when giving a piano lesson to a student who hasn't practiced. I can pray for relief from pain or nausea. I can pray that my cancer doesn't return. I can sense the holiness in my perfectly ordinary life by simply recognizing God's nearness. It is what Jean-Pierre de Caussade refers to as "the sacrament of the present moment." Father de Caussade's belief is mentioned in *The Mystery of Faith*. The author, Father Tadeusz Dajczer, emphasizes that the grace of the moment doesn't come in haste. It comes when there is an awareness that every happening, every suffering, every joy is a sacramental meeting with God.

There are many ways to pray in addition to contemplative prayer as described in Chapter 3. We can pray for our own needs. We can pray for the needs of others. We can pray the prayers of praise and thanksgiving. In a fit of self-pity we might pray the "why me?" prayer. But for me, no prayer is complete without listening time. Good relationships consist of two-way interactions—give/receive and talk/listen. Deepening our relationship with God involves listening. After our talk, our petitions, our complaints, our thankfulness, the time comes to stop and wait in silence and respect to give God time to respond. As Sister Hall mentioned in her explanation of *lectio divina*, sometimes God's response is silence. It is a silence full of meaning, though, leaving us to trust that the meaning will be revealed in time. And it is a silence in which the most fruitful thing we can do is to fully surrender to resting in the peace of God.

I don't know of anyone who can adequately explain why God answers some prayers and not others, why someone being prayed for experiences a miraculous healing and another being prayed for dies. Pastor and religion professor Gerald Sittser explains unanswered prayer as well as anyone I know. He says, "Unanswered prayer breaks us, deepens us, exposes us, and transforms us." Sittser says that if we continue to pray, even though a prayer has been unanswered, we may begin to change *how* we pray and *what* we pray for.

The anonymous author of a commentary in *Forward Day by Day* reminds us that one of the pitfalls of prayer is when we forget which of us is God and which the servant.

As servants we can't test God by giving a to-do list of our wishes, expecting God to take specific directions from us.

In *Praying the Psalms,* Walter Brueggemann suggests that a life of faith doesn't protect us from the pit of despair or grief. "Rather," he says, "the power of God brings us out of the pit to new life, which is not the same as pre-pit existence."

Praying to be cured and praying to be healed are two different things. Author Hawley Todd points out that being cured, in a medical model, is about fixing only one aspect of who we are. On the other hand, healing is a process of bringing all the aspects of who we are into harmony and balance with one another. It is a restoration of wholeness of mind, body, emotions, and spirit. Todd explains that one can be cured without being healed, and one can be healed without being cured.

When we're praying for someone else we need to know the desires of the recipient, lest our prayers conflict with the recipient's prayers. One of our faithful church members had long been struggling with painful cancer and the debilitating effects of her treatments. Her husband of many years died, leaving her lonely, grieving, and distraught. I don't know whether the many people praying for her were praying for her to be cured from cancer or whether they were praying for her to be enfolded in God's love, strength, and comfort. I do know that she reached a point where she refused any further treatments. She was connected with hospice care and sent home where she wanted to die. Since I had taken communion to her on several occasions I knew she was ready to die, with the hope of being with her husband. Being cured was not her wish.

So when we're making intercessory prayers, perhaps for a stranger we've never seen, whose needs we don't know, what do we pray for? How do we pray in a way that is for the highest good of the recipient, a prayer that fulfills the needs of the prayed-for, but doesn't conflict with God's plan? In Paul's letter to the church in Colossae he answers those questions. Paul and his helper-companion Timothy pray that the Colossians "may be filled with the knowledge of God's will in all spiritual wisdom and understanding" (Colossians 1:9). He adds that they are praying for the Colossians to be "prepared to endure everything with patience, while joyfully giving thanks to the Father" (11-12). Those are prayers of healing. Those are prayers that help us to become persons who are whole.

In my years as a psychotherapist helping people through their dying, I came to realize that healing comes in many ways. Sometimes healing is accomplished through dying. Hawley Todd describes healing prayer as a transformative process in which we invite God to be present in our lives. The full significance is that God's presence can transform our earthly life, our dying, and our life beyond death. I try to remember that when I'm praying for someone else.

Persistence in prayer will move us closer to the heart of what God wants for us, rather than what we want or think we should have. Although non-Hodgkin's lymphoma doesn't have a cure, my prayer for myself is for healing—for the restoration of wholeness.

Gerald Sittser explains that God will answer our prayers "in ways that are incomprehensible to us now but will make perfect sense later on when we see the results of God's extraordinary work in our lives." He speaks from personal experience after a tragic accident that killed his mother, his wife, and his young child.

I do know that praying changes the person who is praying. When we "keep on keeping on" in prayer there is a tectonic shift, slow and unobserved, until one day we open our eyes and see that the landscape has changed. We realize our praying has changed, and our prayers have changed.

If cancer is God's way of getting my attention, prayer is God's way of informing and transforming me.

# { 7 }

# CANCER DOESN'T
# HAPPEN TO JUST ONE

I T'S EASY FOR A PERSON with cancer to become self-centered. The many doctor appointments, treatments and scans, and the necessity for rearranging life involves such attention to the needs of the cancer patient that it can be tempting to forget about the needs of others. The toll of cancer, however, embraces a wide world of people who are connected to the patient. This is especially true when the cancer patient lives alone. When a cancer patient lives with another family member, or multiple family members, there is a shifting of responsibilities within the household. There is a different dilemma when a person lives alone, as I do.

The timing of my diagnosis was concurrent with the time to get my income tax report prepared. I have an accountant to prepare my return, but there's always much that I have to do in getting all the figures from the year collected and organized for the accountant. This year I didn't have enough mental and physical energy for the task.

I called my accountant with my problem. It turned out that he had undergone chemotherapy sometime in the past. No sooner had the word "chemotherapy" left my mouth than he replied, "I'll get you an extension." His own experience brought an instant understanding of my plight.

Whether living alone or with other family members the dynamics are shaken when a family member has cancer. This can result in the family becoming closer and more communicative, or it can have the opposite effect of causing disturbing, disruptive behavior among family members. Families who adapt well to change and accept challenges as problems to solve together are the most likely to embrace a member's cancer as a shared situation that involves the input and support of all. The strengths of each member are called upon. The needs of patient, caregivers, and loved ones are interwoven in the fashion of a whole piece of fabric.

Dr. Bernardine Healy, who was herself a cancer patient, commented in her book *Living Time: Faith and Facts to Transform Your Cancer Journey,* "When you're hit with a cancer diagnosis and the ground is getting soft underneath your feet, who and what you love become your anchors." God, my family, my friends, and my church family were my anchors.

In my large, extended family I knew everyone would be concerned and wanting to check on me often. Frequent calls, though, would interrupt the rest I needed. My son Chris volunteered to communicate with all of the family who had access to e-mail. Fortunately, that included most of them. We set up a plan whereby I would immediately contact Chris and Mark after every appointment or treatment or change in my status, and give them the details they wanted. Chris would then send e-mails to all family members. That worked fairly well. It satisfied their need to know and reduced the number of telephone calls I would need to answer.

I knew Chris and Mark were very worried, not only about my health, but also that I might get depressed and anxious. I could tell by their pep talks to me. It was important that I reduce their concern as much as I could. "As much as I hate having this thing," I reassured them, "I'm not depressed. I'm going to get through this." On the other hand, I knew they would want honesty. When I was very sick I didn't soft-pedal my feelings.

My long-time friend Diane offered her assistance as soon as I was diagnosed. When we recognized the need to have someone with me following chemotherapy treatments, I called her. She responded immediately. After the second treatment she left her cats in the care of someone else, drove down from Atlanta, and spent a week taking care of me. She cooked, cleaned, did laundry, and gave moral support and wonderful back rubs. After the third treatment Mark took a week off from his job and flew here from Texas to be my caregiver. He cooked, did the dishes, cleaned up my yard, and did some home repair jobs. He also gave some very good back rubs. I don't think he had ever given a back rub, but he was a natural.

Chris had notified his employer he would take a week off and care for me after the fourth treatment. Fortunately, that treatment turned out to be Rituxan, the maintenance drug, only. Rituxan doesn't have debilitating effects, so I wasn't in need of a caregiver. At a later date Chris brought my grandsons down for a visit, not only to give me some quality time with them, but also for them to see that I was recovering well.

I had hoped I could continue giving piano lessons to my students without interruption. Several of them were preparing for competitions; all needed the continuum. I have always had a mindset that demanded I fulfill my responsibilities, no matter what. "The show must go on," so to speak. Now I experienced being struck down so low that I had to cancel many lessons.

I called all of the parents and explained my situation to them. I gave them the option of what to tell their children. For some the word "cancer" might bring a fear of my death. The mother of a ten-year-old student had died of cancer when the child was only four or five years old. She might have particular problems with my diagnosis. All parents decided not to use the word "cancer." I don't really know what explanation they gave their children. I do know that my students seemed to adapt well to the situation. The parents were very flexible and understanding.

When my hair started falling out I bought a wig. I tried to pick a wig that was close to my normal light brown/gray color and short style. I wanted to look as normal as possible. It didn't fool my students, though. They all noticed a new look. When eight-year-old Andrew walked in for his lesson, he stopped, looked at me carefully, and said, "Is that a haircut or what?"

Andrew later expressed concern for me. His parents obviously had told him only that I was sick. "I've been worried about you," he said. It was important that I reassure him. "I'm doing everything I need to do to get well," I answered. He seemed satisfied with that answer.

During this time I found that my cancer was a vehicle that drove me like a magnet to other people with cancer and formed an immediate bond between us. There's a sense of recognition, almost kinship, like travelers meeting in a foreign country and learning they're from the same hometown. In that situation the conversation starter moves quickly to familiar ground, like "Do you know . . . ?" or "Have you been to . . . ?" or "Where do you go to church?" With cancer the conversation dives right into "Who's your oncologist?" "What kind of cancer do you have?" sort of like a spontaneous support group session.

In preparation for the weekend women's retreat, "A Closer Communion with God," that I was soon to lead, I had contacted a clay supplier to order some clay for use in an experiential exercise. I had never met the man, but he quickly disclosed that his wife had just been diagnosed with an advanced stage of uterine cancer, and he was terribly worried. He obviously had a need to talk. I shared with him my diagnosis and told him I would keep him and his wife in my prayers. After my first treatment made me so sick, I realized I had to cancel the retreat. I called the clay supplier to cancel the order. His wife had just died three days prior to my call. He was devastated and lost. I asked if I could keep praying for him. He replied, "I need all the help I can get."

Kit came to bring communion to me after church one Sunday. She told me she had just been diagnosed with uterine cancer and would have surgery in about a week. Our cancers connected us in a deep understanding of what each of us would be going through. We agreed to pray for each other and stay in touch.

One day I needed to make a copy of some business papers. A friend drove me to an office supply store with a copying center in it. The friend dropped me off in front of the building. While she parked I went into the store to a copy machine. I felt an immediate wave of dizziness and had to lean against the counter with my head lying on top of it to keep from falling. The woman in charge of the copying center came over to me and asked if she could do my copying for me. I gratefully accepted and told her I was being treated for cancer. While she copied my papers she told the story of her husband's cancer. He had gone from being a strong, virile man to one almost helpless from his disease treatments. She recognized in me a member of the community.

My church family became very involved in my healing. At St. Paul's, "church family" takes on its true meaning. Ministering to each other is a strong focus of discipleship that manifests in many ways. With so many people praying for me, I felt it was my responsibility to participate fully in my healing so their efforts wouldn't be in vain.

Soon after my treatments began, Elaine, one of St. Paul's faithful, sent some homemade chicken soup and delicious custard. Later on, she sent more of her good cooking. Many people called to offer help in any way I needed. I knew this wasn't just an obligatory offer. They meant it. Many days I couldn't drive because of fatigue or dizzy spells. One day I called Jean P. to ask her to drive me to an appointment. She responded immediately on short notice and was at my house shortly thereafter. Rebecca, Father Thack's wife, had spent Sunday afternoon with me in the emergency room. Doris called one day to ask when she and Rochelle could deliver a prayer shawl from the prayer ministry. My days were filled with the holiness of ordinary people acting with extraordinary discipleship.

What a precious gift the prayer shawl was! The shawls are knitted by the church prayer shawl ministry and given to those who are going through difficult times. The tag that comes with the prayer shawl reads, "This shawl was handmade. As it was created, we asked God to help you feel his presence and to continue to bless you with courage, strength, hope, and the peace that is beyond human understanding. Please know that we continue to hold you up in prayer and that the warmth of this shawl around your shoulders represents the love we feel for you."

Every morning, except for the days I was too sick to get up, I wrapped myself in the prayer shawl when I began my *lectio divina*. I could feel all of the prayers knitted into the fabric of the shawl as they formed a tapestry with my readings, meditation, and prayers for the day.

All of this ministering from my church family were visible signs that the living Christ is present among us. God has his hands on St. Paul's in a very special way.

I had similar offers from friends and family who aren't a part of St. Paul's, but who also have a Good Samaritan spirit. They always came through when called upon. Often they just volunteered to do things. Rebecca L. and her husband, Neal, spent many hours raking and bagging leaves. Rebecca often drove me to the grocery store, or did the shopping for me. Emily drove me to Mobile and spent an afternoon listening to my piano students play in an honors recital. In addition, she audiotaped the recital for me.

I've always believed in the goodness of people, but the help of all these caregivers was so deep and wide it touched my heart to its core. Never had God been so obviously present.

Living with cancer brings thoughts of our mortality more intensely than ever before. When so many choices are out of our control, we can take charge of our life by planning what we would like to happen at its end. Whether cancer or something else brings its end, making a plan for it will give us the peace that comes from knowing that we have taken care of the loved ones who will survive us. Family members must oversee burial, cremation, or memorial services and the minutiae of business details that are necessary following death; they shouldn't be burdened with having to make so many choices at the time their grief is fresh and raw. As a gift to the ones we love we can make those choices for them and leave the instructions in written form in a safe, readily available place.

On one of my birthdays several years prior to getting cancer, it occurred to me that I should make the plans I desired for the rituals that would occur at the end of my life, even though I was then at the peak of health. If I hadn't already done that, cancer would surely have motivated me to make those plans.

For my end-of-life service I chose the Scriptures, music, and liturgy that have meant the most to me during life. They are on file at St. Paul's and in my bank safe deposit box. Rather than being depressing, the planning was a joyful thing to do. Knowing that when my physical body is no longer here I could share the things I have loved in life with family and friends who survive me has given me a strong feeling of joy. There is an old African proverb, "As long as you speak my name I shall live forever." My favorite music and Scriptures and the prayers I love speak of who I am. Knowing they will be sealed on the hearts of my family and friends gives me a sense of forever being a part of their lives, of leaving a connection that won't be broken.

Taking care of our loved ones before we leave also means leaving clear instructions for them: financial account numbers and passwords; names and contact information for all personal, professional, and commercial organizations we're involved with; names and contact information for friends we want notified upon our death. All of our business transactions should be written and stored in a place easy to access. Several family members should be aware of that place.

Being a survivor of cancer should include the recognition that the people in community with us are also survivors. They have experienced the journey with us emotionally, supported us in our healing, and rejoiced with each victory. If at the end we are healed but not cured, our healing requires that our spirits remain joined with the spirits of our community.

# EPILOGUE

ELEVEN MONTHS AFTER I WAS first diagnosed, a PET scan showed that I was in full remission. This was much earlier than my oncologist had predicted. My voice has returned to its original state, and my hair has grown back. In its new state my hair was curly at first, although it had always been straight until chemotherapy drugs made their mysterious change. Although I was tempted to throw my wig away, I knew I should be realistic and store it in the event I will need it again. I live with that possibility.

God had come bursting into my life anew, in a most ungentle way. God's chosen way shook me into new awarenesses that, in the routine of my life, I probably wouldn't have seen. The familiar paths I walked had become so comfortable that the lenses I looked through had become foggy. Cancer brought the clarity of high definition views.

I have realized that every challenge we face is God working his works through us. It is God stirring our minds to think more deeply, more creatively, more wisely. It is God giving our hearts a chance to awaken to greater generosity, more inclusive love, more openness to all of God's creation, and a deeper understanding of the divine mystery. Sometimes it is God nudging us to be more discerning in our observations and choices. As painful as some of the situations are as we face them, we need to remember that God is in the challenge.

I have learned that faith the size of a mustard seed is enough. As Matthew tells us in his gospel, "For truly I tell you, if you have faith the size of a mustard seed, you will say to this mountain, 'Move from here to there,' and it will move; and nothing will be impossible for you" (17:20).

As any good gardener knows, a seed planted in good soil and nourished faithfully will sprout and grow healthily into what it is meant to be. That is the nature of a seed. Faith, even small faith, will grow when nurtured and will sprout in undetermined and mysterious ways. Faith will help us to grow into the person God wants us to be. As Father John Barr explains in his book *Waylaid by Light,* taking small steps one day at a time will help us to draw near with faith. "Don't wait for full comprehension," he says.

David Douglas, in his *Atlas of Sacred and Spiritual Sites,* comments:

> Nothing . . . can prepare the pilgrim for arrival at the sacred place. Through the preparation and the hardships of the journey, the devotee is opened up to new ways of experiencing. It is precisely this process that transforms individuals and, when they finally arrive at their chosen place, they are in a condition to receive the spiritual benefits of the sacred site and its incumbent rituals. Without the preparation of the journey, the pilgrim is simply a tourist.

As I was told at the beginning of my journey, non-Hodgkin's lymphoma is not a disease for which there is yet a cure. It is a disease that is "managed" or "controlled." I continue to have an intravenous dose of Rituxan once every two months to maintain the remission. This journey hasn't ended. I've learned, though, that trusting in God's unfathomable wisdom and faithfulness to his people leaves me standing on firm ground, even when the winds blow hard. God has been true to his promise to me. Along with the challenges of cancer God remained an unwavering compass, guiding me with the surety of a wisdom greater than anything I could comprehend.

I've been told that chemotherapy treatments leave me more susceptible to other kinds of cancer. I know I must remain alert, with open ears and open mind, to divine messages delivering God's wisdom and will. Good discipleship has eternal dimensions. Today, I'm still a pilgrim with a responsibility to open myself to the meaning and purpose of the journey, so that when I arrive at my destination I am far more than a tourist. I am an experienced traveler, one who has been transformed and made more holy by the journey.

# APPENDIX A

# Choosing Your Medical Team

THE TIME I TOOK TO carefully select a good medical team turned out to be very important. In a situation such as cancer, many things are beyond your control. Choosing the people who will care for you is within your control. Unfortunately, there are some doctors who are brilliant at making diagnoses and prescribing treatments, but who look at a patient as a disease to treat, rather than as a person with real human needs. This isn't the doctor who can give you the emotional support and compassion so vital to someone with a life-threatening illness.

I suggest that you ask many people—both medical and nonmedical—about possible choices. Ask about their experiences with the doctors they recommend. A number of people, including some who had been under his care, highly recommended Dr. Charles Smith, the surgeon I chose to perform my biopsy and, later, to install the port necessary for the infusion of chemotherapy drugs. These were people whose judgment I trust. They were right about the surgeon.

I found the right oncologist by the same method, asking many people who know him. The doctor I chose, Michael Meshad, had not only a fine reputation in the field, but also had been a cancer patient himself. I didn't know him before his cancer, but I believe the experience of walking in the shoes of a cancer patient surely must have helped him to become the compassionate, warm, and caring person that he is. He listened to me, responded to my needs, and patiently answered all of my questions.

I had been a patient of my primary care physician, Suzanne Tormoen, for years and had already developed a trust in her ability as a physician. And when I got my diagnosis of lymphoma she responded, "We're going to help you get through this. If you get anxious, or if you just want to talk or cry, call me." When I went in for appointments she always asked how I was doing emotionally.

Since Dr. Tormoen was a nutritionist before she became a medical doctor, I asked her to suggest foods and drinks that would help build my strength and immunity during the depleting chemotherapy treatments. My refrigerator maintained a large supply of Gatorade and Ensure Plus drinks, as well as eggs, ice cream, chicken, fish, and other high-protein foods.

A pharmacist should also be a part of your medical team. If you choose and use only one pharmacy they will have all your medications in their file. Having all your medications in one place allows the pharmacist to give you valuable and informed help. Once I asked my pharmacist about the comparative effectiveness of Tylenol and Aleve. As soon as I asked she consulted my record on her computer. Seeing that I was on a blood thinner she responded, "As long as you're taking a blood thinner you should not take Aleve."

A home health agency may become part of your team too. Because of the pulmonary embolism I had to take Coumadin (blood thinner) daily. For a time my international ratio (INR) flip-flopped crazily, and I had to have it checked very frequently. INR tells how thick or thin the blood is. At the same time this was happening, I was on chemotherapy and not well enough to drive. A nurse with a home health agency came to my house and checked my INR regularly until it was stabilized. Your primary care physician can connect you with an agency.

# APPENDIX B

# Breathing Exercise 1

THE FOLLOWING EXERCISE WILL PROVE valuable in quieting your mind at the beginning of your Scripture reading and meditation time. It's also beneficial for reducing stress, alleviating pain, and preparing your mind for imagery. It may be difficult to focus your mind at the beginning, but it will get easier once you've learned it. As with learning any new skill, practice enhances your ability to do it.

We can focus on only one thing at a time. If we're focused on our breathing, everything else—stress, anxiety, worries, pain, nausea—will be on the periphery of our attention. In this exercise the goal is to keep your attention on your breathing until it becomes a single-pointed focus. At first, mental chatter will bombard you and take control. Each time that happens, return your attention to your breathing. This will require patience and discipline.

Until you're familiar with the steps, it may be helpful to have a friend or family member read the steps to you *slowly*, giving you plenty of time to follow the instructions. When you're an accomplished breather you'll be able to do this on your own, whenever and wherever you need to.

First, choose a comfortable position, either sitting or lying down. Either way, it's best to keep your back straight. If you're sitting both feet should be on the floor. The goal is to allow your breath to flow freely without the obstacle of a hunched body.

Turn your attention to your breath. At first, just observe your breathing. Initially, it will probably be shallow and perhaps a little fast. Remember that you have the ability to change it.

After you learn what your breath is like, begin to deepen your breathing. Each time you inhale reach deeper down, gradually taking more and more time to draw your breath in. As you exhale feel yourself releasing more and more breath each time. Do this at a pace you find comfortable. As you continue you will find your breath filling your body more and more as you inhale, and releasing more and more as you exhale.

Imagine your breath touching all parts of your inner body, gently massaging muscles, organs, neck tendons, and tissues. Feel your breath moving gently *through* any parts of your body that might be tense or painful. As you exhale allow your breath to release any pain, tension, or other unwanted feelings and symptoms.

Stay focused on your breathing, concentrating on making it deeper and slower. Do not be in a hurry. Be aware of any physical, mental, or emotional changes as your breath slows.

# Breathing Exercise 2

## For Use with Contemplative Prayer

To transition from conscious awareness into contemplative prayer, I begin with Exercise 1. The goal of contemplative prayer is to reach a sense of oneness with God. This requires going to a deeper level of consciousness than is usually achieved in Exercise 1.

One way of reaching the deeper level involves the act of entrainment that I mentioned in Chapter 4. Entrainment occurs when two pulses begin to move in the same rhythm and tempo. Entraining your breathing to the breathing of a loved one brings a great sense of understanding and communion with that person. It's also a fine way to help a person suffering from a panic attack. To do that, match the panicked person's fast, short breaths with fast, short breaths of your own. Then gradually slow and deepen your breathing. The panicked person will involuntarily begin to breathe with you, and become calm.

To attain the desired state for entering contemplative prayer, complete the relaxation steps from Exercise 1. Then imagine yourself matching your breathing with the breathing of Jesus. You may have visual images that arise as that occurs. The image that most often occurs for me is that of Jesus putting his arm around my shoulders and saying, "Walk with me." As we walk I pay attention to his breathing and begin to match my breathing to his. That serves to bring the deep state of silence desired in contemplative prayer—a feeling of resting in God.

I've found this to be a state in which Jesus' promise can be manifested: "But the Advocate, the Holy Spirit, whom the Father will send in my name, will teach you everything, and remind you of all that I have said to you" (John 14:26).

The teachings may not come in words but in silently implanted thoughts and wisdom, or in images.

There are other ways for reaching the deep stillness sought in contemplative prayer. Cistercian priest Thomas Keating has revived the ancient practice of centering prayer. Centering prayer is designed to help you reach the state of interior silence by repeating sacred words, usually words chosen by the person praying. Then there is the "Jesus Prayer" used by some early Christians, i.e., the repetition of "Lord Jesus Christ, have mercy on me." In both of these methods the act of repeating words of worship serves to narrow the praying person's focus and allows him or her to reach the silent and still waiting that is desired. The method most effective for me, however, is matching my breathing to that of Jesus. It arose spontaneously during my daily meditations. I invite you to try it.

# APPENDIX C

## Resources

THE NATIONAL CANCER INSTITUTE (NCI) provides a number of booklets and fact sheets of interest to cancer patients. The publications are free. They may be obtained at:

Telephone:  1-800-422-6237
Internet:    http://www.cancer.gov/publications
Mail:        Publications Ordering Service
            National Cancer Institute
            Suite 3035A
            6116 Executive Boulevard, MSC 8322
            Bethesda, MD 20892-8322

The American Cancer Society's (ACS) publication "Cancer Facts & Figures" contains helpful information. It is free and is updated each year. ACS may be contacted at:

Telephone:  1-800-227-2345
Internet:    www.cancer.org
Mail:        American Cancer Society, Inc.
            250 Williams Street, NW
            Atlanta, GA 30303-1002

Some organizations may give financial help to cancer patients undergoing treatment. For example, the Leukemia & Lymphoma Society gives co-pay assistance to those who qualify. The National Cancer Institute provides contact information on the various organizations.

Contact information for the Leukemia & Lymphoma Society:

P.O. Box 12268
Newport News, VA 23612
1-877-557-2672
www.lls.org/copay

# APPENDIX D

# Lists of Music

THE FOLLOWING ARE LISTS OF music compiled on compact disc programs that I listened to during chemotherapy treatments, plus additional CD programs available commercially. These lists are by no means exhaustive. If you want to do your own search you'll find a world of music that can provide beauty and support for your healing journey.

<u>Emotionally Evocative</u>

Samuel Barber, *Concerto for Violin*, andante

Johannes Brahms, *Double Concerto*, andante

Max Bruch, *Concerto for Two Pianos and Orchestra*, Op. 88a, adagio

Gustav Mahler, *Symphony No. 5, C-sharp Minor*, adagietto

Total time of this program is approximately 35 minutes

<u>Soul Journey</u>

Alan Hovhaness, *Mysterious Mountain*, "Prayer of St. Gregory"

Maurice Durufle, *Requiem, Op. 9*, "Lux Eterna"

Paul Patterson, *Mass of the Dead,* Sanctus

Alan Hovhaness, "Alleluia" from "Alleluia and Fugue"
(fade out at 2:59)

(on same CD as "Prayer of St. Gregory")

Sergei Rachmaninoff, *Vespers* (two selections); "Blessed be the
Man" and "Praise the Name of the Lord"

Maurice Durufle, *Requiem, Op. 9,* "In Paradisum" (on same CD
as "Lux Eterna")


Total time is approximately 30 minutes


<u>Commercially available CDs of calm, meditative music are:</u>


*Baroque Adagios,* Academy of Ancient Music. Decca Records

*Baroque Guitar Favorites,* Gerald Garcia, guitar. NAXOS
Records

*Corelli Concerti Grosso,* Op. 6. Philharmonia Baroque Orchestra

*Morning Mood: The Soft Sounds of Grieg.* Decca Records

*Mozart Adagios.* Ashkenazy, Bell, Hogwood, etc. Decca
Records

*Mozart for Meditation.* Philips Records

*Rachmaninoff: Vespers.* Robert Shaw Festival Singers. Telarc


<u>Music for Healing I</u>, compiled by Ruth Skaggs, available through
www.ruthskaggs.com

# REFERENCES

## Introduction

Kushner, Harold S. 1989. *When Bad Things Happen to Good People.* New York: Schocken Books. 64.

St. Teresa of Avila. 2003. *The Interior Castle.* New York: Riverhead Books. 128.

## Chapter 1

National Cancer Institute. U. S. Department of Health and Human Services. 2011. 1, 5.

## Chapter 2

Metaxas, Eric. 2010. *Bonhoeffer: Pastor, Martyr, Prophet, Spy.* Nashville: Thomas Nelson.

Ornstein, Robert, and David Sobel. 1987. *The Healing Brain.* New York: Touchstone.

## Chapter 3

Dyson, Thack. 2011. "Nothing Like Experience." Sermon presented at St. Paul's Church. 4 Lent, April 3.

Hall, Thelma. 1988. *Too Deep for Words: Rediscovering Lectio Divina.* NewYork: Paulist Press.

Johnston, William. 1976. *Silent Music: The Science of Meditation.* New York: Harper & Row. 18

Metzger, Bruce M. and Michael D. Coogan, eds. 1993. Music and Musical Instruments. *The Oxford Companion to the Bible.* New York: Oxford University Press.

Nouwen, Henri J. M. 1981. *The Way of the Heart: Connecting with God Through Prayer, Wisdom, and Silence.* New York: Crossword Publishing Co. 86.

## Chapter 4

Newham, Paul. 1999. *Using Voice and Song in Therapy: The Practical Application of Voice Movement Therapy.* London and Philadelphia: Jessica Kingsley Publishers. 60-61.

## Chapter 5

Achterberg, Jeanne. 1985. *Imagery in Healing: Shamanism and Modern Medicine.* Boston and London: New Science Library. 3.

Band, Jennie. "The Influence of Selected Music and Structured vs. Unstructured Inductions on Mental Imagery." Ph.D. diss., University of South Carolina, 1996.

Carlson, Linda E. and Barry D. Bultz, "Mind-Body Interventions in Oncology," *Complementary and Alternative Therapies in Oncology* 9 (2008): 127-134.

Gottlieb, Benjamin H. and Elizabeth D. Wachala, "Cancer Support Groups: A Critical Review of Empirical Studies," *Psycho-Oncology* 16 (2007): 379-400.

Horrigan, Bonnie. "Larry LeShan: Mobilizing the Life Force, Treating the Individual," *Alternative Therapies* 1, no. 1 (1995): 62-69.

Kaplan, R. and S. Kaplan. 1989. *The Experience of Nature: A Psychological Perspective.* Cambridge: Cambridge University Press. 173.

Rider, Mark. 1997. *The Rhythmic Language of Health and Disease.* St. Louis: MMB Music, Inc.

Rosenthal, David S. and Elizabeth Dean-Clower. "Integrative Medicine in Hematology/Oncology: Benefits, Ethical Considerations, and Controversies," *Hematology* (January 2005): 491-497.

Skaggs, Ruth. 1997. *Finishing Strong: Treating Chemical Addictions with Music and Imagery.* St. Louis: MMB Music, Inc.

Taylor, Dale B. 1997. *Biomedical Foundations of Music as Therapy.* St. Louis: MMB Music, Inc. 106-108.

Ulrich, R. S. "View from a Window May Influence Recovery from Surgery," *Science* 224 (1984): 420-421.

Chapter 6

Benedict Carey, "Long-Awaited Medical Study Questions the Power of Prayer," *New York Times,* 31 March, 2006.

Brueggemann, Walter. 2007. *Praying the Psalms*. Eugene: Cascade Books. 36.

Dajczer, Tadeusz. 2009. *The Mystery of Faith*. Brewster: Paraclete Press. 42.

*Forward Day by Day*. 2012. Cincinnati: Forward Movement. April 12.

Mytko, Mohanna J. and Sara J. Knight. "Body, Mind and Spirit: Towards the Integration of Religiosity and Spirituality in Cancer Quality of Life Research," *Psycho-Oncology* 8 (1999): 439-450.

Prescott, Bruce. "Science and Prayer and Healing," Oklahoma City. Oklahoma State LPN Association Meeting. (2001) November 13.

Sittser, Gerald L. 2007. *When God Doesn't Answer Your Prayer*. Grand Rapids: Zondervan. 57, 168.

Weaver, Andrew J. and Kevin J. Flannelly. "The Role of Religion/Spirituality for Cancer Patients and Their Caregivers," *Southern Medical Journal* 97, no. 2 (2004): 1210-1214.

Chapter 7

Healy, Bernadine. 2007. *Living Time: Faith and Facts to Transform Your Cancer Journey*. New York: Bantam Books.

Epilogue

Barr, John III. 2008. *Waylaid by Light*. Sumter: Church of the Holy Comforter. 16.

Douglas, David. 2007. *The Atlas of Sacred and Spiritual Sites.* London: Godsfield Press. 37.


Appendix B

Keating, Thomas. 1986. *Open Mind, Open Heart: The Contemplative Dimension of the Gospel.* Amity: Amity House.

www.ingramcontent.com/pod-product-compliance
Lightning Source LLC
Chambersburg PA
CBHW051445280526
45785CB00003B/1433